Medical Marijuana

DR. KOGAN'S EVIDENCE-BASED GUIDE TO THE HEALTH BENEFITS OF CANNABIS AND CBD

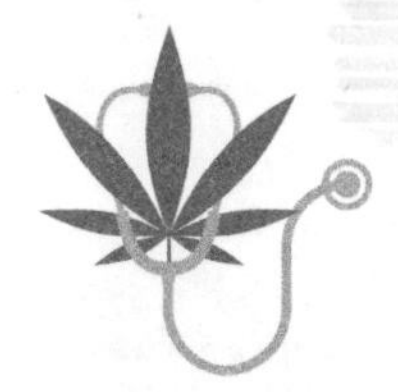

MIKHAIL KOGAN, MD,
and JOAN LIEBMANN-SMITH, PhD

Foreword by Andrew Weil, MD

AVERY
an imprint of Penguin Random House
New York

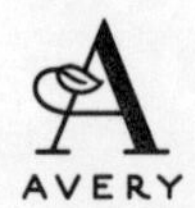

an imprint of Penguin Random House LLC
penguinrandomhouse.com

Illustration on p. 46 by Nenad Jakesevic

Library of Congress Cataloging-in-Publication Data

Names: Kogan, Mikhail, author. | Liebmann-Smith, Joan, author.
Title: Medical marijuana: Dr. Kogan's evidence-based guide to the health benefits of cannabis and CBD / Mikhail Kogan, M.D., and Joan Liebmann-Smith, Ph.D.
Description: New York: Avery, Penguin Random House LLC, [2021] | Includes index.
Identifiers: LCCN 2021017302 (print) | LCCN 2021017303 (ebook) |
ISBN 9780593190234 (hardcover) | ISBN 9780593190258 (ebook)
Subjects: LCSH: Marijuana—Therapeutic use. | Cannabis—Therapeutic use.
Classification: LCC RM666.C266 .K64 2021 (print) |
LCC RM666.C266 (ebook) | DDC 615.3/23648—dc23
LC record available at https://lccn.loc.gov/2021017302
LC ebook record available at https://lccn.loc.gov/2021017303

Printed in the United States of America
1 3 5 7 9 10 8 6 4 2

Book design by Tiffany Estreicher

"There is no room for hypocrisy. Why use bitter soup for healing when sweet water is everywhere?"

"Out beyond ideas of wrongdoing and rightdoing,
there is a field. I'll meet you there.
When the soul lies down in that grass,
the world is too full to talk about."

QUOTATIONS FROM RUMI,
TWELFTH-CENTURY PERSIAN PHILOSOPHER AND POET

To my father, Rudolf, an unrecognized genius who sacrificed his professional career to bring our family to America. To my mother, Zinaida, and my grandmother Shura, who infused into me passion for healing and love of all creatures.

And to the field of integrative medicine and all its champions, advocates, and patients, and to those who believe that nature around us always was, is, and will be a source for healing and transcendent awareness of The Greater.

MIKHAIL KOGAN

To my sister, Susan Handelsman, from whom I learned a lot. Her courage and perseverance have been an inspiration to me.

To the memory of my brother, Peter Liebmann, who died from Parkinson's disease and could have benefitted from medical marijuana had it been legal in his state.

JOAN LIEBMANN-SMITH

Contents

Foreword

Andrew Weil, MD

I was always intrigued by the health benefits of plants and herbs, an interest that led me to become a botany major at Harvard in the early 1960s, when recreational use of pot first appeared on campus. In an introductory course on economic botany, I learned that marijuana (aka cannabis) had been used medicinally for thousands of years. In fact, since ancient times, it's been used to treat myriad conditions, including convulsions, insomnia, nausea, headaches, menstrual pain, and others. However, all that had changed in the United States by the mid-twentieth century; marijuana not only fell out of favor as a medical treatment, it was deemed a dangerous drug and declared illegal.

Because of this designation, researchers in the United States have been prevented from conducting clinical studies into its effects. But as a determined Harvard medical student in the late 1960s, I was able to cut through a great deal of red tape and initiated a small, double-blind, placebo-controlled clinical study on the physiological and psychological effects of marijuana—the first such study allowed to be conducted in the United States. (The Federal Bureau of Narcotics provided confiscated pot for our study.)

Our results were published in 1968 in two leading journals, *Science* and *Nature*.[1] We found that contrary to popular belief, marijuana did not cause the negative effects commonly attributed to it. I was convinced that additional clinical research would also reveal that marijuana was a safe and effective treatment for many conditions, and that it would be legalized within five to ten years. I couldn't have been more wrong! The ongoing designation of cannabis as a Schedule I illicit drug continues to stifle scientific studies in the United States. However, thanks to international research, there is now substantial evidence that it can help treat all the conditions mentioned above, as well as an ever-increasing number of other disorders. More good news is that, in spite of our draconian federal drug laws, marijuana is once again being recognized for its medicinal benefits and is now legal in most states.

The problem is that the internet and bookshelves are flooded with misinformation, questionable testimonials, and false advertising, all of which leave consumers confused and misled. And, unfortunately, most doctors—even those who recommend marijuana to their patients—know very little about it. Dr. Mikhail "Misha" Kogan is a welcome exception; he's one of the few physicians who has expertise in the field of medical cannabis. Since 2012, Dr. Kogan has recommended it to more than three thousand patients and lectured on the subject to countless physicians across the country and internationally. He is the perfect person to convey to consumers the much-needed, evidence-based information they want on medical cannabis. He does that—and even more—in this invaluable book, *Medical Marijuana: Dr. Kogan's Evidence-Based Guide to the Health Benefits of Cannabis and CBD.*

I first met Misha in 2003 when he was a third-year medical student. He came to study at my integrative medicine fellowship program at the University of Arizona as part of his medical school rotations. In addition to taking courses, he worked with me in the clinic. I was impressed with his enthusiasm and exceptionally inquisitive mind. And, importantly, we shared a mutual interest in nature as a source of healing and the belief that the best medicines come from the natural world. Plant remedies—including cannabis—are often safer alternatives to many conventional medications, many of which have potentially serious side effects and may even worsen some conditions over time.

Misha and I have remained in touch ever since his student days. I was pleased that he became an integrative geriatrician—a crucial and neglected specialty. I invited him to become the editor of the first textbook on integrative geriatrics, *Integrative Geriatric Medicine*,[2] which was recently published by Oxford University Press as part of my series of volumes on integrative medicine for clinicians.[3]

I'm now delighted to see that Misha has not only become a leading expert on medical cannabis, but he and his coauthor, medical writer and sociologist Joan Liebmann-Smith, PhD, have written this timely book for consumers on an important subject that is so clouded by misconceptions, misunderstandings, and misinformation. *Medical Marijuana* provides readers with evidence-based information on the health benefits and risks of cannabis, as well as the pros and cons of the different routes of delivery. In addition, readers will find clear explanations of the various forms of cannabis, definitions of the confusing terms, and practical advice on finding certified medical marijuana doctors, reliable dispensaries, and safe products.

Coauthor Dr. Liebmann-Smith provides important historical, political, and sociological perspectives on how marijuana went from being a widely accepted treatment, to being damned as the devil's drug, to its current revival as a legitimate, safe treatment for numerous conditions. The chapters, which contain real patients' stories—as well some amusing and colorful anecdotes—are immensely informative and accessible. *Medical Marijuana* provides readers with the information they need to make educated decisions about using it for their health conditions. It's a must read not only for consumers who are contemplating using medical marijuana for the first time, but also for those who are currently using it and want to expand their knowledge. And, given the gap in knowledge among medical professionals—and the fact that millions of Americans are now using medical marijuana—I highly recommend that doctors, too, read *Medical Marijuana*, not just for their own edification, but for their patients' benefit as well.

Andrew Weil, MD, is the founder and director of the Andrew Weil Center for Integrative Medicine at the University of Arizona, where he also holds the Lovell-Jones Endowed Chair in Integrative Medicine and is a clinical professor of medicine and a professor of public health. He is a best-selling author whose books include Mind Over Meds, Healthy Aging, *and* Eating Well for Optimal Health.

Medical Marijuana

Introduction

Marijuana has been used as a medicine for thousands of years throughout the world. But in the middle of the last century, in the United States and Russia, where I grew up, marijuana became reviled as an evil, dangerous drug. It has since undergone an amazing metamorphosis and is now being hailed as a wonder drug.

I hadn't given medical marijuana much thought until it became legal in 2010 in Washington, DC, where I practice medicine as an integrative geriatrician.[1] More and more patients kept asking me about using it for their medical problems. Many were confused about the benefits and risks; they'd gotten their information—and misinformation—from friends, the internet, and even some doctors.

For my patients' sake, I decided to put aside my preconceptions and delved into the medical literature, which was quite limited. Unfortunately, marijuana is still federally illegal, which has severely hampered research in the United States into its use as a medicine. The good news is that during the past decade, scientists in Israel, Italy, Spain, and other countries have been conducting high-quality research into the benefits and risks of *cannabis* (the scientific term for marijuana) and have published their findings. I read convincing evidence that medical cannabis was safe and effective for treating a wide range of the conditions I was treating, including chronic pain, gastrointestinal problems, sleep disorders, chemo side effects, multiple sclerosis, Parkinson's disease, and even Alzheimer's disease. The conventional medications I was prescribing for these conditions were not very effective, and many of my patients experienced unpleasant and sometimes serious side effects. I started recommending cannabis to a number of them and was astonished at how well it worked, even with some of my oldest patients.

As an integrative geriatrician, I mostly worked with older adults. In fact, my coauthor—medical sociologist Dr. Joan Liebmann-Smith—and I were writing a book on health for seniors. By then, medical marijuana had become legal in most states, and I started to get inundated with calls and referrals from my colleagues who were concerned about the advice their patients were receiving. I began seeing people of all ages who were hoping that medical marijuana would help with their problems.

Medical marijuana's use has since skyrocketed and so has the misinformation about it. Social media, especially, has become flooded with often inaccurate, confusing, conflicting information, and it's difficult for consumers to know what and whom to believe. And, unfortunately, most physicians—even many of those who recommend it to their patients—know very little about the subject. Patients usually wind up having to rely on dispensary staff (aka budtenders)—who are primarily salespeople without medical training—to advise them about what to take for what condition, in what dosage, and by what route. Joan and I realized that there was an urgent need to educate patients of all ages about medical marijuana and decided to write a book that would fill the gaps in their knowledge. Medical marijuana is truly unique; there is no other drug—natural or otherwise—that can treat such a wide range of medical conditions. It's also a complex one; no other drug has so many routes of delivery, combinations of active ingredients, and dosages to choose from.

Medical Marijuana provides readers with reliable, evidence-based information to ensure that they can make wise decisions about using medical marijuana and other forms of cannabis for their medical problems. In the first chapter, "The Long and Winding Road," we describe the convoluted history of medical marijuana from ancient days through modern times, when all the trouble began. The mid-twentieth century was more like the Dark Ages when it came to marijuana. But we've now emerged from the days of "Reefer Madness" into an "Age of Enlightenment," when marijuana has once again regained its rightful place as an effective treatment for a variety of conditions. In Chapter 2, "Cannabis Clarified," we define and explain the very confusing cannabis-related terms, including *cannabidiol, cannabinol, cannabinoids,* and the *endocannabinoid system,* to name a few. We then clarify the confusing and conflicting information about THC, CBD, and the other cannabinoids, especially regarding their benefits, risks, and differing legal statuses. We also cover the importance of terpenes, which give cannabis (and other plants) their unique fragrance and flavor, and the use of cannabis during pregnancy. Chapter 3, "Finding the Right Route," is a practical guide that explains the pros and cons of smoking, vaping, sublinguals, edibles, topicals, and—one of my favorites—suppositories. We also explain which routes of delivery work best for which medical conditions.

Chapters 4 through 9 get to the heart of the matter: we provide evidence-based information and advice on how medical marijuana can help treat aches and pains, sleep and mood problems, GI disturbances, skin disorders, the side effects of cancer treatments, and chronic neurological disorders, including MS, Parkinson's disease, and even Alzheimer's disease. Each of these conditions is illustrated with real-life patients' stories. (Their names and other identifying information has been changed to protect their privacy.) Readers will learn what form of cannabis is best for their particular problem and the importance of following my favorite marijuana mantras: "Start low, go slow," and "Stop when you get to where you need to go."

In the last chapter, "Dealing with Doctors and Dispensaries," we provide practical information on many topics, including how to find a certified cannabis physician who will give you a recommendation for medical marijuana, how to get a medical marijuana ID card, how to choose a dispensary and deal with budtenders, and how to read labels on cannabis products. We also include cost-saving strategies and information about traveling with marijuana, which is still a federally illegal drug. Our appendices include recommended books, websites, online resources; a glossary of terms; and a detailed index.

ROADBLOCKS

While writing this book, we hit some unexpected obstacles: the first was the EVALI (e-cigarette or vaping product use-associated lung injury) "epidemic," which hit the headlines in the winter of 2019. About three thousand mostly young people who had vaped bootlegged cannabis and e-cigarettes that contained vitamin E acetate oil as a thickening agent became very ill, and some even died. But the media made it sound like *all* vaping was dangerous and could kill you. We had to go back and set the record straight so that our readers—who are highly unlikely to use bootlegged vapes—would understand the dangers of vitamin E acetate oil without being deterred from using a form of cannabis that might help them.

As that epidemic died down, the coronavirus pandemic took over. We had to really rethink much of the advice we gave about the potential benefits of vaping (and smoking) pot in these pages and to real-life patients. Although inhaling isn't always my first choice, it did work amazingly well for many of my patients. We now had to focus on the real potential risks of inhaling; COVID-19 can dangerously affect the respiratory system, so anything that can adversely affect our lungs should be avoided. That means inhaling cannabis, especially by older patients and others at high risk. We recommend that they use the other routes of delivery—sublinguals, edibles, topicals, or suppositories—which, in fact, often work better than the inhaled route.

CANNABIS AND COVID-19

There's growing interest—and a lot of hype—about whether cannabis can be helpful in treating or preventing COVID-19. What is currently known is that cannabis does have anti-inflammatory properties, and inflammation is a major driving force in the disease. But research on cannabis for treating or preventing COVID is just beginning, and the results, while promising, are based on lab studies and some animal models, but no clinical (human) studies. Several of these studies have found that cannabis, especially when high in CBD and other cannabinoids and terpenes (see Chapter 2), may be useful in treating COVID when combined with the drugs that have proven beneficial.[2] But more research, especially in humans, is needed to know for sure.

There's also some speculation that cannabis might be helpful for long haulers. At George Washington University, we have established a COVID recovery clinic to try to assist an increasing number of patients presenting with a variety of chronic symptoms. Cannabis can be helpful for some of these symptoms, including insomnia, headaches, chest pain, and numbness or tingling in the arms or legs. Unfortunately, there are usually other serious problems that are even more concerning for patients, such as severe fatigue, shortness of breath, and fast heart rate, for which cannabis is unlikely to be helpful. Until more data is available and providers gain more experience, it's difficult to know exactly what works and what doesn't. But smoked or vaped cannabis should be avoided for any COVID-related problems.

COVID has had another unfortunate consequence: it has affected our collaboration. Although we live in different cities, we found that working together in person was the most productive way to write a book, and we tried to meet as often as possible. But COVID made that impossible. We had to rely on endless emails, copious notes, long phone calls, and multiple Zoom sessions—that is, when we could squeeze them in. As a practicing geriatrician, my patient load exploded with many extremely ill and scared patients. And my wife and I had to spend interminable hours supervising our two young, rambunctious sons' distant learning sessions and homework. Joan was stuck sheltering in place with her husband and geriatric cat in New York, then the epicenter of the epidemic.

MORE ABOUT US

We may appear to be an odd couple: I'm a Generation X geriatrician who grew up in Moscow. Joan is a baby boomer sociologist who grew up in New York. In Moscow, we were taught that marijuana was a dangerous narcotic; if you tried it even once, it would definitely lead you to a world of crime and premature death. When I was in medical school in the United States, marijuana was an illegal drug believed to have no medical merit, so it wasn't part of the curriculum. (It still isn't!) When I started practicing as an integrative geriatrician, I focused on promoting natural, healthy approaches to aging. But because pot was an illegal drug, it was not part of the picture.

Although marijuana was illegal, Joan came of age in a pot-friendly world that not only rejected the *Reefer Madness* mentality but made that movie into a cult film. Plus, she had gone to NYU, which was in the heart of Greenwich Village—the legendary home of hippie culture and potheads. As a medical sociologist, she worked in the field of drug addiction and was keenly aware of the devastation that hard drugs like heroin and cocaine caused. But she also knew that pot was a horse of another color—that it wasn't a dangerous gateway drug. Rather than marijuana turning users into criminals, it was the draconian laws that turned countless people of color into prisoners. Joan was also well aware that, in contrast, middle-class whites could enjoy the pleasures of pot without the fear of arrest. What she was unaware of was the fact that marijuana had medical benefits. In spite of our different backgrounds, we're now definitely on the same page. I came to realize that it's the unfair laws, not the marijuana, that create the criminals, and recommend medical cannabis to many of my patients, including the very elderly.

We've also learned a lot from each other and have had a lot of laughs while writing this book. That's not to say we didn't have our disagreements; in fact, we had many heated discussions and arguments over the use of the word *marijuana*. While we both agreed that we would occasionally use familiar slang terms throughout the book, like *weed* and *pot*, I didn't want the word *marijuana* in the title (see Chapter 2). I preferred the more scientific word *cannabis*. We compromised and used both words.

Our other major argument was over the issue of whether marijuana is an addicting drug, which we discuss at length in Chapter 2. Naturally, we also encourage you to read the rest of the book, or at least the chapters that are relevant to you. We sincerely hope that the information we provide is useful, and that it can help you choose and use medical marijuana in a way that is safe and beneficial for you and your medical situation.

CHAPTER ONE

The Long and Winding Road

Marijuana, which is derived from the *Cannabis sativa* plant, has had a very long, convoluted, and controversial history. In fact, the term *marijuana* wasn't even used until the early twentieth century. Before the mid-eighteenth century, the plant was referred to as *hemp* (or Indian hemp) in English, and by a variety of names across the globe. The ancient Greeks referred to it as *kannabis*, which means canvas, because the plant was primarily used to make cloth. But it wasn't called "cannabis" in English until 1753—when it was officially christened *Cannabis sativa* by the Swedish botanist Carl Linnaeus.[1]

Depending on what part of the plant was used, it was either turned into industrial fiber or consumed for medicinal or other, more controversial purposes. In fact, since ancient times, cannabis has been either revered as a sacred shrub, promoted as a panacea, or damned as the devil's weed.

In just the past one hundred years, marijuana has gone from being a common household cure, to being denounced as a dangerous drug, and finally to being declared illegal. But now it's being resurrected as a wonder weed and, once again, making its way into mainstream medicine. Just how this happened is worth exploring. The past not only can inform us about the potential benefits of medical marijuana, but it also can and should inform medical research. As cannabis researcher and historian Dr. Simona Pisanti explains, "It is surprising that most of the pharmacological properties of Cannabis that only now are being studied were indeed already known and used in medicine for the treatment of numerous pathologies in ancient times."[2]

THE ANCIENT EASTERN WORLD

Medical marijuana's long journey started in ancient China, where archaeologists have dug up evidence that hemp was used for fiber, food, rituals, and medicine as far back as 4000 BCE. Around 2700 BCE, Emperor Shen-Nung described the medical benefits of hemp, called "ma," which were later recorded in the *Shen Nung Ben Ts'ao* (*The Divine Farmer's Classic of Materia Medica*), the world's oldest pharmaco-

ANCIENT ANESTHESIA

Although anesthesia is said to have been invented in Boston in the nineteenth century, almost 1,600 years earlier a doctor in China, Hua Tuo, operated on his patients using mafeisan (boiled cannabis powder) mixed with wine as an anesthetic. Hua Tuo was physician to a tyrannical ruler, Cao Cao, who suffered from terrible headaches. Their doctor–patient relationship didn't end well. According to one legend, Hua Tuo told Cao Cao that he had a brain tumor, which needed to be removed surgically. Cao Cao was furious and accused Hua Tuo of trying to kill him. He not only had Hua Tao beheaded, he had all his medical writings destroyed. It was a double tragedy: Hua Tao lost his head, and the recipe for mafeisan and other cures were lost to history.[3]

peia. Ma was recommended for rheumatism, constipation, malaria, absentmindedness, and "female problems," and was used in childbirth for retained placentas and postpartum bleeding.[4] Not surprisingly, ma had its ups and downs; if used in excess, "ma-fen" (the fruit of hemp) could "produce visions of devils [and on the plus side] over a long term, it makes one communicate with spirits and lightens one's body . . ."[5] Its long-term use was also said to make people fat, strong, and "never senile."[6]

What we now refer to as cannabis spread from China to other parts of the world through trading, migration, and military conquests. It arrived in India around 2000 BCE, and by 1000 BCE, it was considered to be a sacred plant used in religious rituals. "Bhang," as it was called in India, was said to cause happiness, joy, feelings of freedom, and relief from anxiety.[7] It was also used medically as a painkiller, diuretic, anticonvulsive, anti-phlegmatic, appetite stimulant, and aphrodisiac, among other remedies.[8]

ANCIENT MIDDLE EASTERN AND WESTERN COUNTRIES

Since the time of the pharaohs (ca. 3100 BCE), cannabis was used in Egypt for a variety of conditions. The first written evidence, which was found in the *Ramesseum Papyrus* (ca. 1700 BCE), described it as a treatment for eye diseases,[9] while the *Ebers Papyrus* (ca. 1550 BCE) mentioned that it was used to induce childbirth contractions, treat infected fingers and toes,[10] reduce fevers, and heal urinary and rectal problems.[11] It was administered in a variety of ways: inhaled, taken orally, applied topically, and inserted rectally and vaginally,[12] all delivery methods still used today. (See Chapter 3.)

In Israel, archaeologists recently found residues of cannabis that contained THC in an ancient eighth-century BCE temple. This is claimed as the first evidence that ancient Israelis used the drug for

SIBERIAN ICE PRINCESS

Remnants of marijuana were recently found at a 500 BCE burial site in Siberia. They were placed next to a mummy of a young woman dubbed the "Siberian Ice Princess" (aka the Ice Maiden, or Princess Ukok), who was estimated to have been in her twenties when she died. MRIs revealed that the young princess had advanced metastatic breast cancer, but she apparently died from injuries after falling off a horse. Scientists believe that she used the marijuana to help cope with the pain of both.[13] In addition, her mummified skin revealed that her arms, legs, and back were covered with dozens of very detailed, beautiful tattoos.[14] (Given her penchant for pot and tattoos, she would have fit right in at Woodstock!)

religious rituals. In the sixth century BCE, cannabis, which was called "kaneh bosem," was mentioned in the Torah as part of the ritual offerings that Moses gave to God.[15] Almost one thousand years later, in CE 350, kaneh bosem (aka kaneh bosm) was referred to in the Talmud as an intoxicating incense that was burned during religious services.[16]

After taking root in India and Egypt, cannabis spread to Rome, Greece, and other parts of the ancient world. Around 450 BCE, the ancient Greek historian Herodotus described in his book, *The Histories*, how the Scythians of Central Asia would inhale smoke from hempseeds during funerals and "howl in joy."[17] But no mention was made of its medicinal use. Several centuries later, however, the Roman naturalist and historian Pliny the Elder (CE 23–79) wrote about its risks and benefits in his thirty-eight-volume book, *Natural History* (the world's first encyclopedia):

> *Hempseed, it is said, renders men impotent: the juice of this seed will extract worms from the ears, or any insect which may have*

entered them. A decoction of the root in water, relaxes contractions of the joints, and cures gout and similar maladies.[18]

About a century later, the Roman physician Galen wrote that cannabis juice helped relieve earaches, and hempseed cakes could cause hilarity, relaxation, and euphoria.[19] But he also warned that hempseeds were difficult to digest and could hurt both the stomach and head.[20] In the twelfth century CE, Maimonides—the Jewish philosopher and physician to the Egyptian royal court—mentioned that hempseeds and oil were used medicinally, but he didn't provide any details. This may be because by the twelfth century, cannabis had been banned in Jewish and Muslim societies.[21]

THE MIDDLE AGES IN EUROPE

In medieval times in Western Europe, hemp was extensively used to make textiles and other products, but not necessarily for medical purposes. It was, however, a popular folk medicine in Eastern Europe, where it was used to treat toothaches, aid in childbirth, reduce fevers, relieve joint pain, and even prevent convulsions.[22]

An eleventh-century German, Hildegard von Bingen—a nun, herbalist, mystic, composer, and writer—was one of the first Europeans to write about hemp's medical benefits. A true Renaissance woman before the Renaissance, she was also the first woman to write a medical book, *Physica* (translated as *The Book of Medicinal Simples*). She wrote that hemp could help the stomach, wipe out mucus, and relieve pain—especially head pain.[23] As she rather cryptically observed:

Whoever has an empty brain and head pains may eat it and the head pains will be reduced. Though he who is healthy and full of brains shall not be harmed by it. He who has an empty brain shall be caused pain by indulging in hemp.[24]

The medical benefits of hemp became more widely known and accepted in the seventeenth century, when prominent herbalists, botanists, and scholars started writing about its use as a cure for a long list of conditions. In England, in 1640, the royal botanist, John Parkinson, described how cannabis seeds were used to treat intestinal and gallbladder diseases, and how concentrated hemp roots could reduce inflammation and swelling, as well as relieve pain from burns, tumors, gout, and other joint problems.[25] The famous seventeenth-century herbalist and physician-scientist Nicholas Culpeper wrote in his book *Complete Herbal*, "The seed of hemp consumes wind, and by too much use . . . dries up the natural seed of procreation . . . ,"[26] which may or may not have been considered a benefit.

Cannabis wasn't just believed to be useful for physical disorders; the Oxford scholar Robert Burton suggested in his popular book, *The Anatomy of Melancholy* (1691), that cannabis might be helpful for treating depression.[27] About 150 years later, Jacques-Joseph Moreau, a French psychiatrist who is considered the father of modern psychopharmacology, was also interested in the psychoactive effects of cannabis. In the 1840s, he experimented with hashish on himself and his students. Moreau later used it to treat his psychiatric patients and found that it not only helped calm them down, but it also improved their sleep, increased their appetites, and relieved their headaches.[28]

While hashish was all the rage for recreational use, cannabis wasn't very popular for medicinal purposes in Europe at the time. Its big breakthrough came as a result of the careful observations and experimentations of William O'Shaughnessy, a British physician and an army surgeon in India in the 1830s. He was impressed by how the Indians successfully used cannabis as a cure for a number of conditions, which he meticulously documented. He then conducted research studies, first on animals and then on patients—the first cannabis clinical trials in history.[29] O'Shaughnessy found the drug to be both safe and effective: the gold-standard outcome for clinical trials. He reported that hemp extracts and tinctures resulted in the "alleviation

HASHISH HITS FRANCE

Hashish, the highly concentrated and intoxicating resin from the cannabis plant, was discovered by French soldiers during Napoleon's invasion of Egypt in 1798. Because Egypt was a Muslim country, alcohol was banned, but hashish wasn't. The soldiers found it to be an excellent substitute to help them relax and cheer up during downtime. But Napoleon believed that the drug was undermining morale and not only banned its use by the soldiers, but also by the Egyptians.[30] When his soldiers returned to France, they brought hashish home with them along with stories of how paradise could be achieved by just smoking or eating it.[31] Its popularity spread throughout Paris, especially among artists, writers, and other intellectuals. The infamous Club des Hachichins, which was formed in the 1840s, had such illustrious members as Balzac, Dumas, Flaubert, and Baudelaire, who wrote about their sublime experiences.[32]

of pain in most—remarkable increase of appetite in all—unequivocal aphrodisia, and great mental cheerfulness," in all his subjects. And because the drug didn't produce "headache or sickness of stomach," he concluded that "no hesitation could be felt as to the perfect safety of giving the resin of hemp."[33]

When O'Shaughnessy returned to England, he brought a large supply of cannabis with him, and produced and distributed a tincture of hemp, called "Squire's Extract," to other physicians throughout Great Britain.[34] This helped pave the way for the acceptance of cannabis into mainstream medical practice. Based on O'Shaughnessy's research and writing, hemp extracts became widely used during the Victorian era for convulsions, muscle spasms, rheumatism, insomnia, and menstrual cramps, and to induce childbirth contractions.[35] Except for use during childbirth, O'Shaughnessy was way ahead of his time!

It has long been rumored that Queen Victoria used pot for her period pain. And there may be some truth to it; Queen Victoria's personal physician, Sir John Russell Reynolds, was a great champion of cannabis and wrote extensively about its benefits.[36] Two of these benefits—controlling convulsions and relieving nausea and vomiting—are among the most important proven benefits of cannabis today. Also important was Reynolds's recommendation that doctors start their patients on very small doses of cannabis and gradually increase the dose until their patients find relief.[37] As you'll see throughout this book, his good advice is extremely relevant today.

CANNABIS HITS THE NEW WORLD

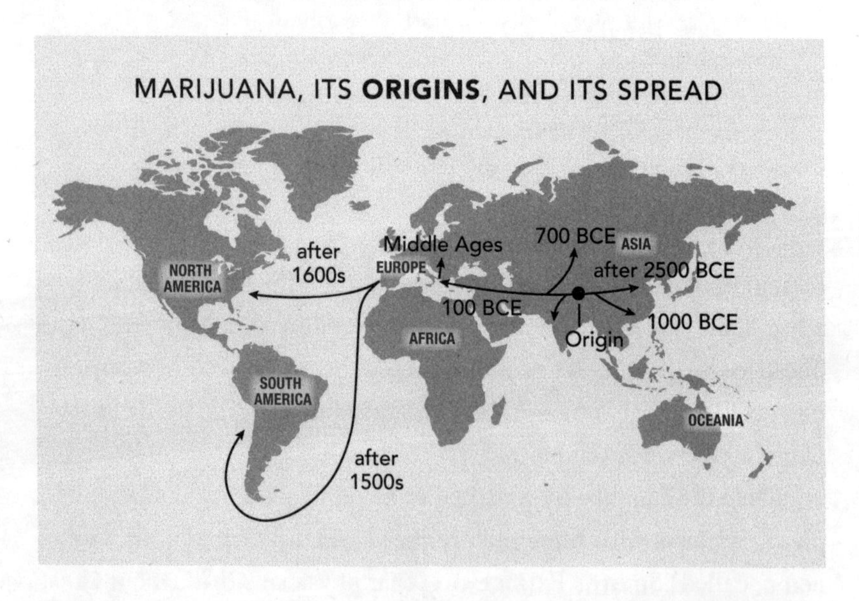

Hemp first arrived in the American Colonies around 1611, when Jamestown settlers brought the plant from England to Virginia to grow for cloth and other products they needed for survival.

England also needed large amounts of hemp, not only for textiles, but for ropes and sails for its military ships. To meet these growing demands, in 1754, King George II offered the American colonists large bounties for sending bales of raw hemp to London. This annoyed Ben Franklin, who complained that there wasn't even enough hemp for the colonists' consumption.[38] Penalties were imposed on farmers who didn't produce the product, and, as a result, hemp cultivation increased dramatically in the colonies to meet the need domestically and abroad and was thus woven into the fabric of our nation. Perhaps if Virginians had discovered some of the other benefits of hemp, they would have come around to approving medical marijuana sooner!

But the medicinal use of hemp didn't really take off on either side of the Atlantic until O'Shaughnessy's publications promoting cannabis as a cure gained traction in the mid-1840s. In 1850, cannabis and its cures were listed for the first time in the United States Pharmacopeia, where it remained until 1942. By the end of the nineteenth century, more than one hundred medical journal articles were published in England and the United States touting the many benefits of cannabis, including for indigestion, poor appetites, migraine headaches, menstrual pain, muscle spasms, insomnia, eczema, gastrointestinal problems, gonorrhea, and even "childbirth psychosis."[39] The 1896 Merck index promoted six cannabis preparations, which were recommended for such conditions as hysteria, tremors, insomnia, gout, depression, and insanity.[40] Anyone could sell it or buy it from apothecaries, general stores, mail-order catalogs, and traveling salesmen. In addition to Merck, other pharmaceutical companies—including Squibb, Eli Lilly, and Parke-Davis—manufactured and sold various forms of cannabis.[41]

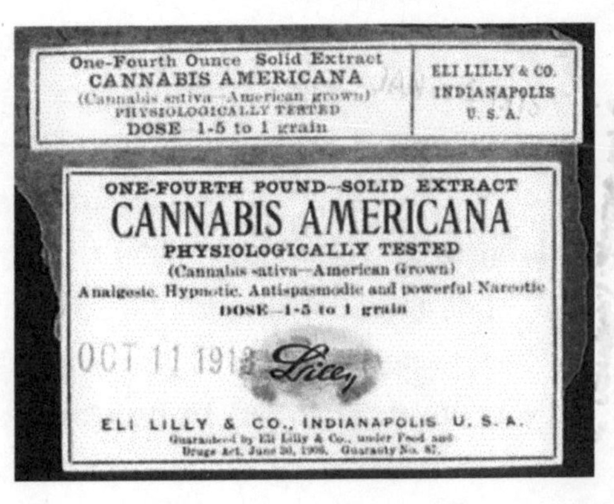

Early Twentieth-Century Eli Lilly Cannabis Label

Cannabis was also considered safer and superior to opiates because it had fewer side effects and wasn't physically addictive. At the turn of the twentieth century, there were a million Americans addicted to morphine or other opioids. Some journal articles even promoted cannabis as a treatment for opiate addiction![42] Talk about history repeating itself: an increasing number of medical journals articles today are providing evidence that cannabis appears to be reducing the use of opioids—and may even help treat opiate addiction.[43] (See Chapter 4.)

So how exactly did marijuana go from being considered an effective, safe cure for many conditions to being maligned as a dangerous drug that leads to madness and even heroin addiction?

THE FALL AND RISE OF CANNABIS

Cannabis elixirs were commonly found in many American households in the late nineteenth to early twentieth centuries, but they soon started to lose popularity. As rival remedies like tranquilizers and painkillers such as morphine, cocaine, aspirin, barbiturates, and hypnotics came on the market;[44] these potent but potentially dangerous drugs won out because they were produced and heavily promoted by the burgeoning pharmaceutical industry. The big game changer came in 1844: the invention of the hypodermic needle followed by the wide availability of injectable morphine. Morphine use shot up in popularity, especially among wounded Civil War soldiers and veterans and other chronic pain sufferers.[45]

It was the Mexican Revolution of 1910, though, that had the biggest hand in the demise of medical cannabis. After the revolution, many Mexicans workers fled to Louisiana, Texas, and other southern and border states, where they were hired and exploited as cheap labor. Some brought *marihuana* (Spanish for Mary Jane) with them, which they smoked for relaxation and relief from their hard labor.[46]

Marijuana then spread to poor immigrant and minority commu-

THE "MEXICAN HYPOTHESIS"

The long-held theory that Mexican immigrants were the cause of the marijuana problem in the United States has recently been debunked by historian Isaac Campos.[47] He claims that marijuana use was not at all common among Mexican immigrants. Many others, including Americans, smoked it. Plus, there was already plenty of crime and poverty in the United States before the Mexicans arrived.

nities at a time when poverty, unemployment, and crime increased. Mexican immigrants, especially, became scapegoats; they were not only blamed for taking jobs away from whites, but for bringing drugs and crime to the United States.[48] Sound familiar?

But it wasn't just the Mexicans who took the heat. In 1911, "Hindoo" immigrants in California became the target of discrimination and were blamed for crime and the spread of marijuana among the white population.[49] In 1913, California became the first state to pass a marijuana prohibition law.[50] Then in 1914, a federal antidrug law called the Harrison Act was passed. However, while it restricted the sale and use of opiates and cocaine, it only imposed a tax on the distribution, sale, or possession of marijuana for nonmedical uses.[51]

With the passage of the anti-alcohol Volstead Act in 1919, prohibition became the law of the land. But it didn't stop people from finding other ways to procure their favorite beverage. Some made their own "moonshine" or "bathtub gin," while others got bootlegged booze at speakeasies or through private connections. Some who couldn't afford to buy it, weren't into DIY brew, or were afraid of getting arrested or poisoned by adulterated alcohol found another alternative. Smoking "weed" or "reefers" became a cheaper, easier, and safer option. "Tea pads" soon became the rage in large cities—especially in Black and other minority neighborhoods—where "hepsters," jazz

MARIJUANA MUSIC

In the 1920s and '30s, smoking reefers became popular among both Black and white jazz players. "Reefer songs," which were recorded by leading jazz musicians including Louis Armstrong, Cab Calloway, and Benny Goodman, became big hits in the 1930s.[52] Another big hit at the time was "La Cucaracha" ("The Cockroach"). Originally a battle song of the Mexican Revolution, it was made famous by Judy Garland—along with her sisters—who sang it in Spanish in one of her earliest movies, *La Fiesta de Santa Barbara.*[53] The lyrics in English—*"The cockroach, the cockroach, cannot walk anymore because it hasn't, because it lacks marijuana to smoke"*—were rarely understood. In fact, "La Cucaracha" is still very popular among schoolchildren in the United States, but perhaps with different lyrics.

musicians, artists, radicals, and freethinkers could hang out, get high, and listen to the newly popular reefer music.[54]

THE DARK AGES

During Prohibition and the Depression, tea pads were not considered a big problem, much less a threat to society. But Black people, Mexicans, and other immigrants were. Many were demonized in the belief that they were having sexual relationships with white women. They were also accused of giving drugs to young children and blamed for lost jobs and increased crime. These alleged social problems were based on racism but attributed to reefer smoking.[55] The anti-marijuana campaign intensified, and sensational articles started appearing describing these alleged horrible crimes.

The success of the temperance movement's fight against alcohol encouraged marijuana opponents to jump on the bandwagon and

REEFER MADNESS

The now infamous film *Reefer Madness* hit theaters in 1936. While in those days it may have helped turn people away from turning on, *Reefer Madness* became a cult classic with hippies in the '70s, who watched the movie stoned! The film is still popular as high entertainment today.

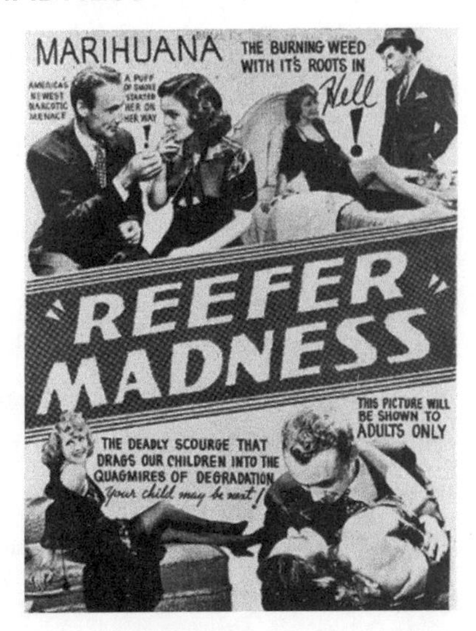

launch a massive campaign against the "killer weed" and the growing "marijuana menace." It was felt that the public had to be hit hard with something frightening enough to turn them off marijuana. The answer: scary posters and a horror film, *Reefer Madness*.

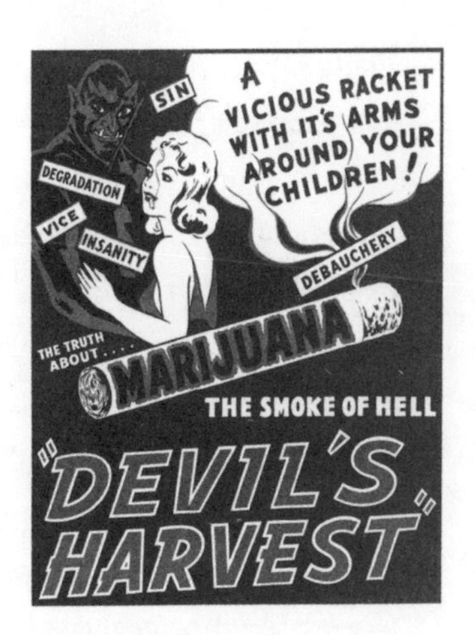

1936 Movie Poster

In 1937, Harry Anslinger, head of the Federal Bureau of Narcotics (FBN), pushed hard for a new law, the Marijuana Tax Act, which would be the government's first attempt to criminalize marijuana. But by then it was a moot point: all forty-eight states had already passed laws against the use of marijuana.[55]

In defense of the law, Anslinger testified before a US House committee that:

Most marijuana smokers are Negroes, Hispanics, jazz musicians, and entertainers. Their satanic music is driven by marijuana, and marijuana smoking by white women makes them want to seek sexual relations with Negroes, entertainers, and others. It is a drug that causes insanity, criminality, and death—the most violence-causing drug in the history of mankind.[57]

Anslinger also contended that marijuana was a "gateway drug" that would lead to heroin use and addiction. Ironically, the one major opposition to the proposed Marijuana Tax Act came from the American Medical Association (AMA). The law required that a doctor who prescribed marijuana reveal the patient's name, address, and diagnosis—a clear violation of the doctor/patient relationship. They also objected to the medical misinformation used to justify the act and issued a major report stating that:

There is positively no evidence to indicate the abuse of cannabis as a medicinal agent or to show that its medicinal use is leading to the development of cannabis addiction. . . . There is a possibility that a restudy of the drug by modern means may show other advantages to be derived from its medicinal use. (Journal of the American Medical Association, 1937)[58]

The AMA report couldn't have been more prescient. As we describe below and throughout this book, research has indeed found that cannabis has many significant medical benefits.

Congress ignored the AMA's objection and passed the Marijuana Tax Act in 1937. Although the tax was small ($1.00 per year in most cases), the penalty for doctors, patients, and others breaking the law was enormous, up to $2,000 in fines and five years in prison, or both![59] The act also removed cannabis from the 1942 US Pharmacopeia—where it had been listed since 1850.

Opponents of the act started doing their own medical and socio-

CANNABIS FOR CANARIES

The AMA wasn't the only group testifying against the proposed law; the producers and distributors of birdseed complained that canaries would not sing as well—or might stop singing altogether—if marijuana seeds were eliminated from their diet. Congress acquiesced and amended the bill allowing the production and sale of sterilized birdseed that couldn't be reproduced.[60] Clearly canaries had more clout than the AMA and marijuana users. While canaries could happily sing for their supper, cannabis consumers could wind up in Sing Sing!

logical research to disprove the feds' claims of the dangers of marijuana. The popular outspoken mayor of New York, Fiorello La Guardia, commissioned the prestigious New York Academy of Medicine to study the issue. Their research findings, "The Marihuana Problem in the City of New York," was published in 1944, directly refuted virtually all the claims made by the feds. The academy reported that marijuana was *not* physically addicting, did *not* lead to crime, and was *not* a gateway drug that led to heroin or cocaine use and addiction.[61] Angered by the report, Anslinger rejected their conclusions, declaring that the report was unscientific or—in today's parlance—fake news.

Rather than easing up on laws, the feds doubled down. In 1951 and again in 1956, bills were passed that imposed mandatory minimum sentences for all marijuana offenses; even first-time offenders received from two to ten years in prison.[62]

The law failed as a deterrent. During the 1960s marijuana was not only a mainstay of the beatniks and hippies, but rapidly gained popularity among the average middle class. By 1970, 42 percent of college students smoked pot, as well as more than half of US soldiers in Vietnam.[63] President Richard Nixon was determined to do something about the growing menace. In 1970, he signed the Controlled Substance Act (CSA) into law. Under this act, cannabis was designated a

Schedule I drug, which made it federally illegal. The CSA determined that cannabis, like heroin and LSD, had a high potential for abuse, was dangerous, and had no therapeutic benefits. (Interestingly, cocaine, morphine, and amphetamines were considered less dangerous than marijuana and, therefore, only classified as Schedule II drugs.) Rather than having a dampening effect on marijuana *use*, the Schedule I designation only stifled cannabis *research*—a consequence that still reverberates today.

Nixon felt a still more aggressive approach was necessary to deal with the problem and declared a "War on Drugs," stating that drug abuse was "public enemy number one." As recorded in an official transcript of the May 26, 1971, Oval Office meeting between Nixon and his chief of staff, H. R. Haldeman, Nixon—not one to mince words—said to Haldeman:

> *I want a Goddamn strong statement on marijuana. . . . I mean one on marijuana that just tears the ass out of them . . . every one of the bastards that are out for legalizing marijuana is Jewish. What the Christ is the matter with the Jews, Bob, what is the matter with them? I suppose it's because most of them are psychiatrists. . . . By God we are going to hit the marijuana thing, and I want to hit it right square in the puss.*[64]

In spite of Nixon's unorthodox anti-Semitic rantings, there was a brief hiatus in the War on Drugs from the mid- to late '70s. In 1972, the Nixon-appointed Shafer Commission came out with a report that recommended that the possession of marijuana be decriminalized. As a result, eleven states decriminalized the possession of small quantities of marijuana.[65] Nixon wasn't pleased, dismissed the findings (more fake news), and pushed for even more marijuana arrests and stricter penalties. He kept up his crusade to criminalize marijuana until 1974, when he was forced to resign or face impeachment and criminal charges. The new president, Gerald Ford, wasn't as freaked out about marijuana as his predecessor. In fact, he ordered a review to see if the current laws were actually effective.[66] He might have been influenced by the fact that his twenty-three-year-old son had recently admitted to smoking pot and said that it should be treated like alcohol.[67] Ford defended his son, but not the legalization of pot. He did, however, put more of an emphasis on fighting heroin use than marijuana use.[68]

When Jimmy Carter ran against Ford for president in 1976, one of his major campaign pledges was to decriminalize marijuana. He won, and during the first year of his presidency, possession of up to one ounce of marijuana was decriminalized.[69] But the respite didn't last long. After Ronald Reagan won the presidency in 1981, he doubled down on the War on Drugs, and his wife, Nancy, launched her antidrug campaign, "Just Say No." Then, in 1986, the Anti-Drug Abuse Act was passed, which reestablished mandatory minimum jail sentences for certain drug offenses. Three years later, President George H. W. Bush declared a new War on Drugs at the local, state, and federal levels, calling for more prisons, jails, courts, and prosecutors.[70] When Bill Clinton became president, he emphasized the importance of testing and treatment of drug abusers to cut down on the imprisonment of addicts.[71] He also famously admitted he had smoked pot as a student, but "didn't inhale."

Since the Clinton administration, nothing much has changed regarding the nation's drug policy. But the incarceration rate for drug offenders continued to increase dramatically; it jumped from 41,000 in the 1980s to 440,000 in 2018.[72] And Blacks are six times more likely to be imprisoned for drug crimes than whites.[73] Astoundingly, an average of 1.5 million people a year, most of whom are Black men, are arrested merely for the possession of pot.[74]

This turns out to be not very surprising. More than forty years after Nixon declared his War on Drugs, his real motives were recently revealed by John Ehrlichman, Nixon's chief counsel. In an interview with journalist Dan Baum, which was published in the April 2016 issue of *The Atlantic*, Ehrlichman said:

> *You want to know what this was really all about? . . . The Nixon campaign in 1968, and the Nixon White House after that, had two enemies: the antiwar left and black people. You understand what I'm saying? We knew we couldn't make it illegal to be either against the war or black, but by getting the public to associate the hippies with marijuana and blacks with heroin, and then criminalizing both heavily, we could disrupt those communities. We could arrest their leaders, raid their homes, break up their meetings, and vilify them night after night on the evening news. Did we know we were lying about the drugs? Of course we did.*[75]

THE NEW AGE OF ENLIGHTENMENT

While the United States was in the drug dark ages, demonizing marijuana and imprisoning tens of thousands of mostly people of color merely for the possession of pot, science was trumping politics in more progressive countries, especially in Israel. In the early 1960s, Dr. Raphael Mechoulam, a young Israeli biochemist at the Weizmann Institute in Rehovot, decided to pursue research into the biological properties and effects of cannabis. Mechoulam, now considered the Father of Cannabis Research, had read numerous nineteenth-century papers touting the benefits of cannabis and wanted to see if their findings held up to today's standards.[76] This is a perfect example of how history can inform research. In 1964, Mechoulam and his colleague Dr. Yechiel Gaoni discovered and synthesized THC, the main psychoactive component of cannabis.

He and his colleagues continued their research and several years

CANNABIS FROM COPS

The only way the Father of Cannabis Research, Dr. Raphael Mechoulam, was able to procure cannabis for his research was through a connection who put him in touch with the head of the investigative branch of the Tel Aviv police station. According to Mechoulam, "I obtained 5kg of superb, smuggled Lebanese hashish. I took a bus back to Rehovot, nobody in the bus realizing that the smell from my bag was from hashish. Later we found that both the head of the investigative branch of the police and I had broken quite a few laws."[77] Mechoulam revealed that more than forty years later, he was still getting hashish for his research from the police.

later discovered additional *cannabinoids*, the term Mechoulam coined for the active components of cannabis. More than one hundred cannabinoids have now been discovered. In 1992, two scientists in Mechoulam's lab at Hebrew University—Dr. Lumír Hanuš and his American colleague, Dr. William Devane—discovered the existence of cannabinoid receptors in our bodies, which form the basis of the endocannabinoid system (ECS). The ECS is a major body system that affects every organ and cell in our bodies, from our brains to our reproductive systems, and is responsible for maintaining our health. These important discoveries, which are explained in Chapter 2, helped provide the scientific evidence for the therapeutic benefits of cannabis.

Without Mechoulam and other scientists' breakthrough research, we might still be in the cannabis dark ages. Their groundbreaking discoveries were catalysts for countless other scientists around the globe to study the biology and benefits of cannabis and publish their results. But little, if any, of this research has been conducted in the United States.

ROADBLOCKS

Our restrictive, racist, counterproductive, outdated drug laws still continue to severely hamper cannabis research in the United States. The insistence that cannabis is a Schedule I drug—and therefore federally illegal—interferes with clinical research that could shed more light on the benefits and safety of medical marijuana, important information for consumers.

Still, good news travels fast and encouraging results from abroad prompted states to rethink their anti-marijuana laws. In 1996, California, which had been the first state to criminalize marijuana, finally redeemed itself by becoming the first state to legalize medical marijuana. Since then, the majority of states have joined them. As of publication, thirty-six states and the District of Columbia have legalized medical marijuana.[78] Nineteen of these states also have legalized recreational marijuana. While hopes are high that more states will follow, the journey from *Reefer Madness* to mainstream medicine still has a ways to go. The endless fight against legalization continues, and the pharmaceutical industry has had no small role in this battle.

The pharmaceutical industry has managed to bypass the federal law against marijuana as far back as the 1980s. Several companies got FDA approval to manufacture synthetic THC (Marinol and Cesamet) and, more recently, cannabis-derived CBD (Epidiolex), all of which are legally sold by prescription today. (See Chapter 2.) As was pointed out in a recent Emory University law article, it's the height of hypocrisy that the feds made marijuana illegal off claims that it was harmful and without medical benefits, only to grant approval for these pharmaceutical cannabis products with similar risks and benefits.[79]

As you will read later in this book, these prescription (Rx) pharmaceutical drugs do have benefits for such conditions as chemo-related nausea and vomiting, poor appetite, some forms of epilepsy, and multiple sclerosis spasticity, among others. And they also have the same side effects as natural cannabis. However, they're extremely expensive and not well tolerated, or even liked, by consumers. Medical cannabis sold through dispensaries not only has the same benefits but contains other important components missing from pharmaceutical cannabis, especially terpenes, which give marijuana and other plants their flavors and aromas. These and other natural ingredients enhance the effects of cannabis, a phenomenon known as the "entourage effect." (See Chapter 2.)

So why would patients pay hundreds if not thousands of dollars for these Rx drugs when they can buy more reasonably priced medical marijuana in dispensaries or even grow it in their own backyards? This conundrum has pitted the manufacturers of these synthetic and cannabis-derived drugs against cannabis farmers and distributors.

Lobbyists for pharmaceutical companies also have a vested interest in fighting the legalization of medical marijuana, and they're aggressively doing just that,[80] partially by keeping consumers in the dark by preventing clinical research into the benefits of medical marijuana by keeping it a Schedule I drug.[81] There's also increasing evidence that medical marijuana users are substituting it for prescription opiates, barbiturates, antidepressants, and anti-anxiety and other conventional prescription medications. This is referred to as the "substitution effect,"[82] which we describe in the upcoming chapters.

But there is some good news on the legal front: the passage of the 2018 Farm Bill made industrial hemp and hemp-derived CBD federally legal. It set 0.3 percent THC as the dividing line between hemp and marijuana. If cannabis-derived hemp contains more than 0.3 percent THC—which it often does—it's designated federally illegal. Most hemp products as well as CBD contain only trace amounts of THC, though, so they can be legally sold to consumers.[83] The catch-22 is that although these products are legal, it's illegal to market them as therapeutic agents unless they have previously been approved for those purposes by the FDA—something they make exceedingly difficult to do.[84]

Another obstacle to legalizing medical marijuana is the stigma attached to its use. Many politicians, physicians, consumers, and even researchers still believe marijuana is a dangerous drug that has no medicinal value. But these stigmas are disappearing because of the publication of hundreds of articles demonstrating that medical marijuana can be helpful for a long list of conditions. In addition to the ones mentioned above, it can help relieve chronic pain as well as reduce some skin, GI, mood, and sleep problems, among others discussed in this book. Surveys have found that not only are more patients using medical marijuana to help with these problems,[85] but large numbers of doctors believe it can help their patients suffering from them.[86] At long last, marijuana users have morphed from being labeled criminals to being recognized as legitimate patients.

And speaking of stigma, in an amazing reversal of fortune, Mexico has gone from being vilified as the initial source of the marijuana problem in the United States to potentially becoming the largest supplier of legal marijuana in the world![87]

Marijuana's trip on its long and winding road is finally winding down. In spite of all the roadblocks, the journey from *Reefer Madness* to mainstream medicine may be closer than ever to reaching its goal.

CHAPTER TWO

Cannabis Clarified

Cannabis is not only a highly controversial topic, but also a very confusing one. For example, marijuana, hashish, hemp, cannabis, cannabidiol, cannabinol, and cannabinoids are closely related, but they all have different meanings, chemical compositions, biological effects, and legal statuses.

Cannabis is a member of the *Cannabaceae* family, a small family of flowering plants that includes about 170 species. Interestingly, two of the most famous family members of the *Cannabaceae* family, *Cannabis sativa L.* (hemp) and *Humulus lupulus* (hops), give us marijuana and beer, respectively. Although their lesser-known third cousin, *Celtis occidentalis* (hackberries) is by far the most prevalent member of the family, it doesn't have the same appeal—or kick—as its cousins.

Before we get into the definitions and details of the confusing cannabis-related, tongue-twisting terms, we'll try to tackle the most commonly used, misused, and controversial term for cannabis: *marijuana.*

WHAT IS MARIJUANA?

Marijuana (aka marihuana) continues to be the most common term for cannabis. As we explained in Chapter 1, both the word and the recreational use of the drug were introduced to the United States after the Mexican Revolution in 1910. Biologically, marijuana and cannabis are the same thing. They refer to the parts or products of the *Cannabis sativa* (hemp) plant containing at least 0.3 percent tetrahydrocannabinol (THC). THC is the ingredient responsible for the psychoactive (mind-altering) effects—especially the high—associated with pot.

To further confuse matters, the term *cannabis* is sometimes misused in reference to the cannabis plant, not the drug. Cannabis refers only to products derived from the cannabis plant that contain 0.3 percent or more THC, not to products that contain less, such as cannabidiol (CBD) or hempseed.

To clarify things, throughout this book we use the term *cannabis plant* when specifically referring to the plant itself rather than the actual drug, cannabis. Also, we use the terms *cannabis* and *marijuana* interchangeably. We'll explain why later in this chapter (see "The M-Word Controversy" below). For variety's sake, we also use such popular terms as *pot, weed, grass,* and *flower.* All these names refer to products derived from the cannabis plant and, as we mentioned above, contain at least 0.3 percent THC. This percentage is also an arbitrary cutoff point for determining the legal status of cannabis plant derivatives and products. As we discussed in Chapter 1, in 1970 the FDA declared that any form of cannabis, and any cannabis-derived product that has more than 0.3 percent THC, should be designated as a Schedule I controlled substance and is, therefore, federally illegal. Since the passage of the 2018 Farm Bill, some forms of cannabis, such as CBD and industrial hemp that have less than 0.3 percent THC, can be legally bought in most states.

HASHISH

Hashish is a substance derived from the resin of the cannabis plant that generally has much higher levels of THC than marijuana. It's used primarily recreationally for its intoxicating effects and is typically smoked, vaped, or eaten. The American writer Alice B. Toklas was the first to cook up hashish brownies and put the recipe in her famous 1950s cookbook. Hash brownies soon became a rage among hippies in the 1960s.

To add to cannabis confusion, there are many different species, strains, and varieties of cannabis. Botanists have long divided cannabis into three distinct species, *sativa, indica,* and *ruderalis,* but this distinction is now being challenged.

THE CANNABIS-STRAIN CONTROVERSY

Both *Cannabis indica* and *Cannabis sativa* were first identified in 1793. *Sativa* is the larger of the two plants and has a higher concentration of THC. Historically, it's been considered stimulating and energizing and best used during the day. *Indica,* on the other hand, is considered calming and best used in the nighttime. As we explain below, these claims are now contested.

Cannabis ruderalis, the new kid on the block, was only identified in 1924. It's considered the runt of the litter because it's the shortest and skinniest and contains the least amount of THC. Although it can't get you high, it does have a high concentration of CBD and is believed to have a calming effect. However, it's not very popular or widely available in dispensaries.

To further complicate things, hybrids have become major players. As the term implies, hybrids are a combination of different strains of cannabis. Because of hybridization, there are now countless varieties of cannabis available, each with a different level of potency and effects.

Cannabis experts now claim that the standard classification of cannabis as *sativa* or *indica* is outdated and obsolete. Recent research has revealed that there really is no meaningful distinction between them. It's not the plant's size or shape that makes a difference in whether weed is sedating or stimulating. Rather, other factors come into play, especially the ratio of THC to CBD.

However, when you walk into any medical or recreational dispensary, you will find that almost all products list *indica*, *sativa*, or hybrid on their labels. While I have no doubt that in the future, most classifications will be more precise and include other cannabinoids and terpenes (see below), listing indica and sativa can be useful. While most people will find *sativa* stimulating and *indica* relaxing, there are some who have paradoxical reactions and experience the opposite effects.

THE ABCS OF THC AND CBD

THC (delta-9-tetrahydrocannabinol) is the psychoactive ingredient in cannabis, commonly referred to as marijuana, pot, weed, and grass, to name a few. As we mentioned in Chapter 1, THC was first discovered and synthesized in Israel in the early 1960s by Dr. Raphael Mechoulam, who is considered the Father of Cannabis Research, and his colleagues. In addition to its intoxicating effects, THC has anti-inflammatory, anti-anxiety, and analgesic effects. In spite of these proven benefits, cannabis products that contain more than 0.3 percent THC are Schedule I, federally illegal drugs and can only be obtained in states that have legalized medical or recreational marijuana.

THC flower is the most popular form of marijuana and comes from the sticky or hairy reproductive parts of the female cannabis plant called "trichomes." Cannabis flower is high in THC and usually smoked or vaped. But other forms of THC can be eaten, placed under the tongue, applied to the skin, or inserted as suppositories. Each delivery method has its pros and cons (see Chapter 3).

There are several cannabinoids that are related to THC, most notably THCa and THCV, which are less popular but also appear to have some important medical benefits.

THCa (tetrahydrocannabinolic acid) is a nonintoxicating cannabinoid found in the raw cannabis plant. It's actually the precursor to THC. It's only when the cannabis plant is activated by heat or light (called "decarboxylation") that THCa converts to THC and becomes psychoactive. That's why you can get high from smoking or vaping, but you won't get high if you eat fresh, raw cannabis leaves or flower. Researchers are just beginning to study the effects of THCa, and the preliminary results have been encouraging. It appears to have anti-inflammatory, neuroprotective, anti-seizure, anti-nausea, and analgesic properties, among other potential benefits.[1] The best way to consume it is through THCa tinctures or edibles, which are made from raw cannabis. Because THCa has a strong, bitter taste, mixing raw cannabis juice with fruits or vegetables has become increasingly popular. It's also legal in most states.

THCV (tetrahydrocannabivarin) is an offshoot of THC that's considered a minor cannabinoid because it's found in only some cannabis strains, often in trace amounts. There's debate as to whether it's a psychoactive drug because its effects vary by dose. At low doses, THCV is not psychoactive and can actually inhibit the intoxicating effects of THC. But at high doses it can boost those effects.

There have been only a few research studies on the health effects of THCV, but so far they have had positive results. There's preliminary evidence that THCV may be helpful in reducing epileptic seizures as well as some of the symptoms of schizophrenia.[2] It may also help boost the anti-inflammatory, anticancer, and analgesic effects of other cannabinoids.[3] Other studies have found that THCV might be helpful in treating diabetes as well as chemotherapy-related nausea

LEGAL LUNACY

Because THCa is not designated as a Schedule I controlled drug, it can be legally sold in most states. It can then be heated and converted to THC, even in states where THC is still illegal. This doesn't make sense and is very confusing to patients and physicians alike. That had been the case in Virginia, where I practice, until spring 2021 when THC was legalized. Patients who had medical cannabis cards could obtain THCa from dispensaries but not any product containing THC. So those who want to get high could just heat up THCa by smoking or vaping it, or baking with it, thus turning it into psychoactive THC. There wasn't a week that went by that I didn't get an email from an enthusiastic patient or a doctor saying how happy they were that Virginia had finally approved THC! I had to burst their bubble and tell them that they still couldn't get any THC products at Virginia dispensaries. Many patients might not be willing to go to the extreme of heating THCa to get an unpredictable dose of THC that could make them very high or have other side effects, when all they want to do is get some pain or nausea relief from a reliably produced THC product. These legal drug distinctions and decisions highlight the complete folly of drafting state drug laws without the critical input of cannabis specialists. Luckily, Virginia had the good sense to finally end the lunacy and approve THC. High five, Virginia!

---

and vomiting.[4] And while THC can give you the munchies, THCV appears to suppress appetite, and so it might be useful for treating obesity.[5] There's also evidence that it could be a promising treatment for Parkinson's disease.[6] Although it's not illegal, THCV can be difficult to procure because it's usually found only in trace amounts in most cannabis strains, but higher quantities can be found in some South African *sativa* strains and in some hybrids.

Delta-8 THC, another form of THC, has recently become a hot item, with exploding sales, especially in states that haven't yet legalized marijuana. Sometimes referred to as "marijuana lite," Delta-8 doesn't produce the same punch as THC, but many people find that it's a good way to get a legal, albeit milder high. It comes in a variety of forms, including vapes, tinctures, gummies, and even lotions. Except for its weaker psychoactive effects, Delta-8 is very similar to THC (i.e., Delta-9 THC). The National Cancer Institute describes Delta-8 as an "analogue of tetrahydrocannabinol (THC) with antiemetic, anxiolytic, appetite-stimulating, analgesic, and neuroprotective properties . . . (but) with lower psychotropic potency."[7] However, it's the high, not health, that motivates most users. Whether Delta-8 does, in fact, have any medical benefits is unknown because it's been studied even less than THC.

Also unknown is Delta-8's legal status: whether it's legal is an ongoing, heated debate. Because THC is derived from cannabis, it's definitely a Schedule I, federally illegal drug. Delta-8, however, is purported to be legal because it's typically derived from hemp, which was made legal with the passage of the 2018 Farm Bill (see "Roadblocks" in Chapter 1). That said, the US Drug Enforcement Administration (DEA), which determines the legality of a drug, has designated Delta-8 as an illegal Schedule I drug.[8] But that might soon change. The DEA is now in the process of reexamining the 2018 Farm Bill, which would include reviewing regulations over Delta-8 and other forms of marijuana. In the meantime, Delta-8 remains in legal limbo. According to a DEA spokesperson, the DEA "would be unable to comment on any impact in legality of tetrahydrocannabinols, delta-8 included, until the process is complete. We are in the process of reviewing thousands of comments and do not speculate on what could happen as a result."[9]

CBD (cannabidiol) has now become as popular, if not more so, than THC. It's the nonintoxicating compound derived from the cannabis plant; it only contains trace amounts (less than 0.3 percent) of THC. CBD can be derived from either marijuana or hemp.

Marijuana-derived CBD is federally illegal if it contains more than 0.3 percent THC, which it often does. Because hemp-derived CBD has less than that, it's not classified as a Schedule I drug and, therefore, is widely available legally in stores and on the internet. But there still are some restrictions on how it's labeled and advertised (see Chapter 1). Another issue is that because hemp contains very little CBD, it often takes many plants to extract an adequate amount. This increases the risk of contamination with toxins and pollutants. There's also no real quality control over the production of hemp-derived CBD, and there have been many reports of poor-quality products. Marijuana-derived CBD usually has better quality control. The downside is that it's only available in cannabis dispensaries and can be quite expensive. Hemp-derived CBD is not only cheaper, it's also legal in most states and can be bought in a variety of stores and on the internet.

In general, CBD has anticonvulsive, anti-inflammatory, antioxidant, antipsychotic, anti-anxiety, and neuroprotective effects. As we mentioned above, CBD has also been shown to help counteract the high of THC—a plus or minus, depending on the user. It's important to be aware that CBD can also interact with other drugs, increasing the risk of side effects as well as interfering with their effectiveness.

IS CBD REALLY NOT PSYCHOACTIVE?

CBD is often described as being nonpsychoactive, but experts disagree. Their argument goes that because it has antipsychotic, antidepressant, and anti-anxiety effects, it is definitely psychoactive.[10] According to Rachel Knox, MD, medicine cannabis expert and activist:

> *As medical scientists it's about high time that we acknowledge, once and for all, that all cannabinoids are psychoactive in their own ways, albeit to different degrees. This includes CBD. They just aren't intoxicating like THC. . . . Psychoactivity speaks to a*

substance's ability to affect cognition, behavior, mood, motor activity, perception, awareness, consciousness, etc., most, if not all, of which CBD can do.[11]

There are several cannabinoids related to CBD that are also legally available. Their effects and potential benefits are described below:[12]

CBDa (cannabidiolic acid) is the botanical precursor of CBD, similar to the way that THCa is a precursor to THC. CBDa is found in raw cannabis plants and only becomes CBD when heated. There's evidence that it can have important benefits for such conditions as epilepsy, anxiety, and chemotherapy-induced nausea and vomiting. It's also been shown to kill certain cancer cells in animal and lab studies. In addition, CBDa is a potent anti-inflammatory and analgesic, more potent per milligram than such NSAIDs (non-steroidal anti-inflammatory drugs) as Motrin and Advil. This is especially important because NSAIDs are not only some of the most commonly used drugs but also have potentially serious—or even life-threatening—side effects. Another benefit is that, unlike CBD, CBDa does not interact with other drugs, thus making it safer than CBD.

CBC (cannabichromene) is a promising nonintoxicating cannabinoid. Similar to THC and CBD, it has anti-inflammatory and analgesic effects and may be useful in treating inflammatory bowel disease (IBD). It also has sedative, anti-anxiety, and antidepressant effects, and may counter the intoxicating effects of THC. In addition, it appears to have antifungal and antibacterial properties.

CBN (cannabinol) is a close cousin to CBD. It has anti-inflammatory, analgesic, and anticonvulsive effects. It also has mild psychoactive effects and can act as a sedative, especially when used with THC. In fact, it has the most sedative effects of all the cannabinoids, so it is an excellent choice for sleep problems. Other possible benefits include appetite stimulation, the promotion of bone growth, and a treatment for glaucoma and psoriasis.

CBG (cannabigerol) is a nonintoxicating cannabinoid that has been shown to reduce pain and inflammation. It also holds promise as an appetite stimulant and a treatment for some gastrointestinal problems, mood disorders, and neurological conditions. Even more impressive is that, according to some animal studies, it's able to inhibit the growth of certain cancers.

As a geriatrician, I'm very excited about the potential use of CBG as a safe and effective appetite stimulant for older adults, and I'm in the middle of planning a small clinical trial to test this hypothesis. I've also seen CBG effectively used when combined with CBD and THC to treat inflammatory skin disorders such as chronic eczema.

Just how THC and CBD can be beneficial for so many different conditions is explained by another groundbreaking and truly remarkable discovery in 1964 by Dr. Mechoulam and his colleagues: the endocannabinoid system.

WHAT IS THE ENDOCANNABINOID SYSTEM?

The endocannabinoid system (ECS) is a major body system that encompasses every cell and organ in our bodies, from our brains to our reproductive organs. It appears to be an ancient system that exists in most animals. The ECS plays an important role in regulating almost all aspects of our metabolism, hormones, and nervous system. It's

CANNABIS QUOTE

"By using a plant that has been around for thousands of years, we discovered a new physiological system of immense importance. We wouldn't have been able to get there if we had not looked at the plant."[13]

—Dr. Raphael Mechoulam

involved in digestion, sleep, emotions, fertility, memory, immunity, and pain sensitivity, among other vital functions.

In the late 1980s and early 1990s, scientists discovered what makes the ECS tick. It turns out that it's made up of a collection of cannabinoid receptors that are located throughout our bodies. Cannabinoid receptors are like tiny locks on the surface of cells, and cannabinoids are the keys that can unlock them and tell them what to do. The two main cannabinoid receptors are CB1 and CB2, and it's through these receptors that the ECS is able to regulate the key body functions mentioned above.

CB1 receptors are found predominantly in the brain and spinal cord and are responsible for pain control, coordination, cognition, emotions, and other central nervous system functions, as well as being responsible for the well-known marijuana effects.[14] CB2 receptors, on the other hand, are located in almost all other systems, but they can also be found throughout the nervous system. CB2 receptors appear to be most concentrated in the immune system, which controls inflammation and protects many physiological systems from injuries and infections.[15]

Interestingly, THC binds with both CB1 and CB2 receptors, which is why and how it can produce therapeutic effects. While CBD doesn't attach to either receptor, it interacts with THC in several important ways. When added to THC, CBD can decrease THC's psychoactive side effects while increasing its nonpsychoactive benefits. CBD also plays a key role in helping to keep our ECS in balance.

Researchers wondered why our bodies had cannabinoid receptors that could only be activated by THC—something we could only get from a plant. They believed that this made sense only if our bodies also produced its *own* cannabis. Mechoulam and his coworkers soon discovered that the ECS does indeed make its own "cannabis." Because they're made inside our bodies, these compounds are called "endocannabinoids." (*Endo* is Latin for "inside.") In other words, scientists discovered that we make our own version of marijuana. And legally at that!

The best way to understand how endocannabinoids work is to think of them as internal keys that our bodies produce that can unlock CB1 and CB2 receptors, which then help our ECS keep functioning well and our bodies healthy. But sometimes the keys get lost, stuck, or stop working altogether. This is where THC comes in. THC is like an external master key that we can use when internal keys get rusty. It fits very neatly into those tiny locks to get our ECS and bodies functioning properly again.

In addition to producing similar effects in our bodies as cannabis does, endocannabinoids are critical to our health because they maintain homeostasis in the ECS. When our bodies don't produce enough,

---

DISCOVERY OF FIRST ENDOCANNABINOID

The first endocannabinoid was discovered in 1992 by two members of Dr. Mechoulam's lab at Hebrew University: Lumír Hanuš and William Devane. Because it binds to the same receptor (CB1) as THC and has the same psychoactive effects, they named it "anandamide," which is a play on the Sanskrit word for supreme joy or bliss. Anandamide is not only the first endocannabinoid discovered but arguably the most important one and the most abundant.

---

we can suffer from wht Dr. Ethan Russo calls "endocannabinoid deficiency." According to Dr. Russo, a world-renowned expert in cannabis and the endocannabinoid system, when we don't have enough endocannabinoids, the ECS becomes imbalanced and our key body systems malfunction. We then suffer the consequences with a variety of disturbing symptoms, including chromic pain, digestive disorders, and insomnia, to name a few. As Dr. Russo further explains:

> *If you don't have enough endocannabinoids, you have pain where there shouldn't be pain. You would be sick, meaning nauseated. You would have a lowered seizure threshold. And just a whole litany of other problems. . . . [A] number of very common diseases seem to fit a pattern that would be consistent with an endocannabinoid deficiency, specially these are migraine, irritable bowel syndrome, and fibromyalgia.*[16]

This is when THC can come to the rescue. As we mentioned above, THC can activate CB1 and/or CB2 receptors. By doing so, it can fill the gap and help restore balance in the ECS and relieve unpleasant symptoms.

It's not just THC that plays a key role in dealing with endocannabinoid deficiencies. Other cannabinoids can also help, especially when combined with THC.

WHAT EXACTLY ARE CANNABINOIDS?

There are actually three types of cannabinoids, all of which can produce therapeutic and other effects:

1. Endocannabinoids: As we described above, these are natural cannabis-like compounds produced inside the human body,

which are the key components of the endocannabinoid system. They can have the same physiological and psychoactive effects as cannabis when they activate certain receptors.

2. Phytocannabinoids: These popular cannabinoids are derived from the cannabis plant and sold in dispensaries. Of the more than 100 phytocannabinoids identified so far, THC and CBD are the most well-known and medically important ones. Although THC is still federally illegal, it can now be legally obtained in a growing number of states with a doctor's recommendation, and CBD is legal in most states. Phytocannabinoids are natural plant-derived products and are usually referred to as just cannabinoids. They shouldn't be confused with synthetic cannabinoids, which are also often simply called cannabinoids but are totally different.

3. Synthetic cannabinoids: These are pharmaceutically developed drugs that mimic the effects of natural cannabinoids, are FDA approved, and are available only by prescription. These man-made drugs include dronabinol (Marinol) and nabilone (Cesamet), which are approved for chemotherapy-related nausea and vomiting, and as an appetite stimulant for AIDS and cancer patients.

To further confuse matters, the term *synthetic cannabinoids* also refers to synthetically made—and often toxic—street drugs such as K2 and Spice. This "fake weed" is a far cry from the FDA-approved synthetic cannabinoids, yet they share the same name, which may be the reason that many journal articles now refer to FDA-approved synthetic cannabinoids as just cannabinoids. However, this makes it difficult to interpret results of studies because we don't always know what drugs they're actually referring to: FDA-approved pharmaceuti-

CANNABIS-DERIVED PHARMACEUTICALS

In 2018, Epidiolex (cannabidiol) became the first natural form of cannabis to be approved by the FDA. This CBD extract is effective for the prevention of seizures in children and adults who have very rare, severe forms of epilepsy. Another naturally derived cannabis, Sativex (nabiximols), contains both THC and CBD. It helps control neuropathic pain and some multiple sclerosis symptoms. However, as of publication, Sativex is not yet approved by the FDA.

cal cannabinoids or the phytocannabinoids sold in dispensaries. To simplify the matter, we'll usually refer to these drugs as Rx pharmaceutical cannabinoids or synthetic pharmaceuticals.

Because pharmaceutical cannabinoids have limited use and are very expensive, we'll focus on phytocannabinoids, which are by far the most widely available and popular cannabinoids for medical as well as recreational use. They're also natural and reasonably priced. And, depending on the state you live in, phytocannabinoids may be sold in marijuana dispensaries. Also, patients overwhelmingly prefer them to pharmaceuticals, which not only have more side effects, but often don't work very well.

Regardless of what they're called, both natural and pharmaceutical cannabinoids have been proven to have benefits for a host of medical conditions, including chronic pain, nausea, and vomiting from chemotherapy; multiple sclerosis spasticity; and some sleep and anxiety disorders, among others.[17] There are countless other benefits that have been reported but not adequately studied (or at all), since clinical research on the benefits of cannabis has been severely restricted because of our drug laws. That said, botanists, chemists, and other scientists are uncovering many more wonders of weed. They're looking into the physiological and therapeutic effects of THC, CBD, and their offshoots, as well as how different cannabinoids can work together to enhance those effects (see "The Entourage Effect" below), which are further enhanced by terpenes. More than 150 different terpenes have been identified in cannabis plants.[18]

WHAT ARE TERPENES?

Terpenes are a large group of oils found in cannabis and other plants; they're responsible for a plant's distinctive aromas, flavors, and therapeutic effects. Cannabis terpenes are produced by trichomes—microscopic mushroom-shaped, hairlike growths that protrude from the buds and flowers of the female cannabis plants. Although terpenes can be found in cannabis, CBD, and hemp essential oils, the concentration of terpenes is higher in cannabis essential oils.[19]

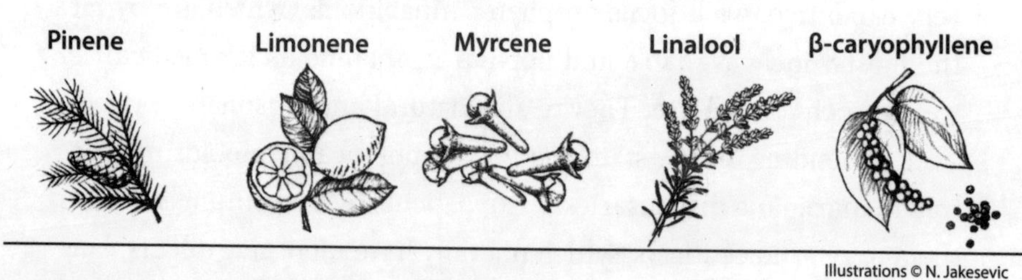

Aroma: Pine
Effects: anti-inflammatory, antiseptic, antibacterial, gastroprotective, anticancer

Aroma: lemon, citrus
Effects: anti-inflammatory, antioxidant, sedative effects, gastroprotective

Aroma: cloves, earthy
Effects: sedative, muscle relaxant, analgesic, anticancer

Aroma: lavender, sweet citrus
Effects: sedative, anti-anxiety, anti-depression, anti-inflammatory, analgesic

Aroma: Black pepper, woody, spicy
Effects: sedative, anti-anxiety, anti-depression, antioxidant, anticancer, anti-inflammatory

The following are the most popular and important terpenes found in the cannabis plant:[20]

Pinene (pine) has anti-inflammatory, antibacterial, antiseptic, gastroprotective, and anticancer effects. It can act synergistically with CBD to help relieve pain and may be useful for

CANNABIS QUOTE

"The healing power of cannabis most likely resides in terpenes/terpenoids and phytocannabinoids, of which particular compounds, their amount, and the ratio to each other play the most important role in the treatment of particular diseases."

—Lumír Hanuš, a leading authority in cannabis research who codiscovered the first endocannabinoid[21]

treating osteoarthritis. It's also been shown to increase alertness and improve memory. Pinene may also be helpful for treating asthma.

Limonene (lemon, citrusy) has anti-inflammatory, antioxidant, gastroprotective, and sedative effects. It can enhance the anti-stress and anti-anxiety properties of CBD. It may also help treat asthma and osteoarthritis. There's also evidence that limonene can act as a chemo-preventive agent and has been shown to kill lung cancer and breast cancer cells in animal studies.

Myrcene (cloves, earthy) has been used throughout history as a painkiller. Mycrene can enhance the analgesic effects of THC and CBD, as well as the anti-inflammatory effects of CBD. It's a potent sedative and muscle relaxant. It has been shown to improve glucose tolerance and may be helpful in treating diabetes. Myrcene also appears to have anticancer effects.

Linalool (lavender, sweet citrus) has sedative, anti-anxiety, and antidepressive effects, especially when combined with CBD. It's been used for centuries to treat insomnia. Linalool also has anti-inflammatory and painkilling properties. Used topically, it appears to help treat skin burns without leaving scars. Linalool has shown promise in preventing convulsions.

β-caryophyllene (BCP) (peppery, woody, spicy) is an antioxidant and anti-inflammatory that can combat pain and insomnia. It also enhances the analgesic and anti-inflammatory effects of THC and may be helpful in the treatment of gastrointestinal problems, diabetes, anxiety and depression, and multiple sclerosis. It's been shown to have some anticancer effects.

THE ENTOURAGE EFFECT

As you can see, the positive effects of THC and CBD can be greatly enhanced by specific terpenes. In 1998, Dr. Mechoulam dubbed this phenomenon the "entourage effect." According to this concept, the different components of the whole cannabis plant—such as THC, CBD, and terpenes—work together synergistically to produce better and longer-lasting therapeutic benefits. In other words, the sum is greater than the parts.

With all the potential benefits of the related forms of THC and CBD mentioned above, how does one choose what to use? The good news is you don't have to. That's the beauty of whole-plant extracts.

ARE WHOLE-PLANT EXTRACTS, FULL-PLANT EXTRACTS, FULL-SPECTRUM EXTRACTS, AND BROAD-SPECTRUM EXTRACTS THE SAME THING?

As you probably realize by now, nothing in the cannabis world of words is simple, and this is no exception. *Whole-plant extracts* and *full-spectrum extracts* are exactly the same thing; all the active ingredients in the whole cannabis plant are extracted to produce them. So in addition to THC and CBD, whole-plant cannabis extracts contain a variety of cannabinoids, including THCa, THCV, CBDa, CBG, and CBN, as well as terpenes and other active ingredients. When combined, they produce—you guessed it—the entourage effect. As a result, their therapeutic benefits are enhanced. Whole-plant CBD oil is similar to whole-plant cannabis extracts, but it only has trace amounts of THC. To confuse matters even more, there are *full-plant extracts*. They go through less processing than whole-plant or full-spectrum extracts and so have more natural ingredients, including vitamins, fibers, and other nutrients.

Finally, there's *broad-spectrum extracts* (aka broad-spectrum CBD oil), which is similar to whole-plant CBD oil except that *all* the THC has been removed.

Now that you've conquered those convoluted terms, we want to introduce you to two more: *FECO* and *RSO*.

WHAT IN THE WORLD ARE FECO AND RSO?

FECO (full-extract cannabis oil) is basically the same thing as whole-plant extract in oil form. It's one of the most commonly used and effective preparations for a whole host of conditions covered in this book, including pain, inflammation, and poor sleep, among others.

FECO is made by extracting the active ingredients of cannabis flower and transferring them to oil, which can then be carefully measured and ingested or applied. It's not only the best of weed in a small bottle, FECO provides a very high potency cannabis that can be delivered in a variety of ways other than smoking or vaping. For example, it can easily be used sublingually or as a base for topical applications or rectal and vaginal suppositories, or even cooked into brownies or made into ice pops.

RSO (Rick Simpson Oil) is another full-spectrum cannabis oil

FECO FIRST

FECO is arguably one of the most versatile and useful forms of medical cannabis. It's the one I most frequently first recommend to my patients for a variety of conditions. It's also almost always available in dispensaries. If you can't find it, it probably means that your dispensary is more geared to recreational rather than medical marijuana. Raise hell and head for another dispensary!

that is much higher in THC and/or CBD than other full-spectrum oils. It's named after Rick Simpson, a Canadian cannabis activist and engineer who found that the oil helped relieve the severe symptoms he developed after a bad accident. He was later diagnosed with skin cancer, and the oil helped cure that as well.[22] In contrast to FECO, RSO has a much higher concentration of THC, often 90 percent or even higher!

Unfortunately, if the oil extraction is done incorrectly, which has happened in the past, it can lead to contamination and an inferior product. The good news is that as more and more producers engage in correct extraction methods, high-quality RSO is becoming more widely available. This is especially good news for the increasing number of cancer patients who are using RSO along with their standard cancer treatment. RSO has also generally had one of the lowest costs per milligram compared with other THC extracts. I like recommending RSO when high doses of THC/CBD need to be delivered in one dose. For example, RSO can be used as a base for suppositories for people with severe back pain who need quick relief. Suppositories provide a good alternative option when high doses are needed. (See Chapter 3.)

DO ISOLATES HAVE ANY BENEFITS?

While there are enormous benefits to whole-plant extracts, isolates can also have a therapeutic role to play. That's why the pharmaceutical industry is so keen on developing isolates. Sativex is a good example: it's a cannabis isolate containing THC and CBD that is used for various pain disorders (see sidebar above, "Cannabis-Derived Pharmaceuticals"). While approved in Europe, it has not yet been approved by the FDA for use in the United States.

I mostly recommend whole plants or whole-plant extracts for my patients, which they prefer anyway. In my experience, patients find that isolates have more side effects and are less effective. This is most likely because of the entourage effect in whole-plant extracts. Not only can they be more effective than isolates, but less THC is needed to obtain the desired therapeutic effect, so there are fewer side effects.

DOES MEDICAL CANNABIS HAVE ANY PROVEN BENEFITS?

In 2017, the National Academies of Sciences, Engineering, and Medicine released their landmark report, "The Health Effects of Cannabis and Cannabinoids: The Current State of Evidence and Recommendations for Research."[23] The report, which was based on reviews of abstracts of more than ten thousand scientific studies, found that the evidence was conclusive or substantial that:

> *Cannabis or cannabinoids are effective for the treatment of pain in adults; chemotherapy-induced nausea and vomiting and spasticity associated with multiple sclerosis. Moderate evidence was found*

for secondary sleep disturbances. The evidence supporting improvement in appetite, Tourette syndrome, anxiety, posttraumatic stress disorder, cancer, irritable bowel syndrome, epilepsy and a variety of neurodegenerative disorders was described as limited, insufficient or absent.[24]

More recently, in 2020, the American Heart Association (AHA) published a report of their own literature review of the risks and benefits. Below is a summary of what they found to be the proven, possible, unproven, or inconclusive benefits of cannabis and/or CBD.[25]

PROVEN OR POSSIBLE BENEFITS

- Reduce pain (including fibromyalgia, neuropathic, and cancer pain)
- Reduce multiple sclerosis pain and spasticity
- Reduce nausea and vomiting caused by chemotherapy
- Increase appetite and weight gain in cancer and HIV/AIDS patients
- Reduce seizures in epilepsy
- Reduce long-term opioid use and withdrawal symptoms
- Reduce dystonia (uncontrollable muscle contractions and movement common in Parkinson's disease and other neurological disorders)

UNPROVEN OR INCONCLUSIVE BENEFITS

- Reduce anxiety and depression
- Improve sleep
- Reduce symptoms of Crohn's disease and ulcerative colitis
- Reduce Alzheimer's disease symptoms

While compelling, these findings about the proven or unproven benefits of cannabis and other cannabinoids aren't written in stone—nor are they inclusive. Although they're based on the reviews of thousands of studies, these studies are conducted in many countries using different methodologies, patient populations, and forms of cannabis, among other key variables. The effects of cannabis depend on a web of important factors, especially drug composition, doses, and delivery routes, all of which make generalizing about the pros and cons of cannabis problematic at best. And there are many other reported benefits that have not been widely studied. Benefits, in fact, are often in the eyes of the beholder. There's an enormous trove of compelling testimonials and anecdotal evidence from both physicians and patients about the beneficial effects of different forms of cannabis or cannabis-derived products that shouldn't be discounted. That said, some testimonials, especially those on commercial cannabis internet sites, that seem too good to be true probably are. Still, patient success stories are what drive—or at least should inspire—good clinical research.

WHAT ARE THE QUALIFYING CONDITIONS FOR MEDICAL MARIJUANA?

Doctors in states with legalized medical marijuana cannot "prescribe" it, they can only "recommend" its use to patients who have a qualifying condition. And each of those states has its own list of qualifying conditions. According to a recent large survey of medical marijuana patients in twenty states and Washington, DC, the most common qualifying conditions they reported were chronic pain, multiple sclerosis muscle spasms, chemo-induced nausea and vomiting, post-traumatic stress disorder, and cancer. Other qualifying conditions mentioned in order of frequency were epilepsy, loss of weight and appetite, inflammatory bowel disease, HIV/AIDS, glaucoma, dementia, and arthritis.[26] It's also up to each state as to which doctors are qualified to recommend medical marijuana to their patients. Some states require the physician to be certificated, but few states require these doctors to take a cannabis course.[27] Physician surveys indicate that most doctors don't feel that they are knowledgeable enough to counsel their patients.[28] This gap in knowledge can be a serious problem for patients who count on their physicians for information about the benefits and potential risks of medical marijuana (see Chapter 10).

WHAT ARE THOSE POTENTIAL RISKS?

As with any drug, cannabis products have some potential adverse effects. They can be very mild to quite severe and depend on a number of variables; these include dosages, delivery routes, added ingredients, length of use, and individual risk factors, among others.

Any smoked or vaped cannabis can cause respiratory problems, including wheezing, chronic cough, bronchitis, and even lung damage, especially among heavy users.[29] This is of special concern because of the recent EVALI (e-cigarette or vaping product use-associated lung injury) and COVID-19 epidemics (see Chapter 3). The good news is that cannabis does *not* cause lung, head, or neck cancer, even when inhaled.[30]

In general, CBD and CBD products have fewer serious side effects than THC. That said, there have been reported side effects from CBD, which include drowsiness, fatigue, mood changes, reduced appetite, dry mouth, diarrhea, and allergies, especially skin allergies. In addition, high dosages have been linked to liver damage and reduced fertility in men.[31] Also, as mentioned above, one of the main concerns about CBD is its interaction with other medications, either increasing or decreasing their effects.

One of my older patients overdosed on oxycodone (a prescription opioid) after a relative suggested he take a high dose of CBD capsules with the opioid to help relieve his pain. His wife called me to say she was concerned because he had become very lethargic. She would

CANNABINOID HYPEREMESIS SYNDROME

Paradoxically, cannabis has been implicated in a rare, recently discovered disorder—cannabinoid hyperemesis syndrome (CHS)—which primarily affects young pot users who are heavy, chronic users. This bizarre condition—first reported in 2004—is characterized by cyclic bouts of uncontrollable vomiting and severe stomach pain, and—even more bizarrely—a compulsion to take hot showers or baths.[32] Unfortunately, conventional antiemetics don't work well. And while long, hot baths or showers and capsaicin cream on the abdomen may temporarily relieve the symptoms, the only cure is total abstinence from marijuana.[33] Cannabinoid hyperemesis, which only occurs in humans, may be the result of a toxic buildup of cannabis.[34] There have also been an increasing number of cases caused by the use of synthetic, nonprescription cannabis, such as K2 and Spice.[35]

wake him up and have him drink some water, but he'd fall right back to sleep again. I asked her if he had been taking any new medications or supplements, and she said he had taken CBD capsules in addition to the oxycodone. I told her he should immediately stop the CBD and not take oxycodone for twelve hours. Luckily, he rebounded to his usual self within forty-eight hours and was able to resume taking oxycodone—but no CBD! If he had continued taking it, he would have ended up in the hospital, or worse—dead.

However, compared with CBD, THC has considerably more—and potentially more serious—side effects. In addition to the respiratory problems mentioned above, other adverse effects include the following:

1. Central nervous system (CNS) problems: Cannabis can cause dizziness, euphoria, cognitive impairment, paranoia, hallucinations, and psychosis.

2. Cardiovascular problems: Cannabis can increase blood pressure and palpitations. The American Heart Association just published a study on the cardiovascular effects of cannabis. They concluded that there was compelling evidence that cannabis—especially when smoked or vaped—increased the risk of cardiac problems, including heart attacks and heart failure.[36] They recommend that people not smoke or vape cannabis (or other substances) because it can damage the heart, blood vessels, and lungs.

Consuming too much cannabis at once can cause any of the above problems, and in some cases can even lead to an overdose. The signs of a cannabis overdose are similar to the adverse effects but more severe. According to the CDC:

> *These signs may include extreme confusion, anxiety, paranoia, panic, fast heart rate, delusions or hallucinations, increased blood pressure, and severe nausea or vomiting. In some cases, these reactions can lead to unintentional injury such as a motor vehicle crash, fall, or poisoning.*[37]

CANNABIS AND CAR CRASHES

Other potentially serious CNS cannabis side effects are space and time perception changes, which have been linked to an increase in car crashes. So it's just as important to heed the message "Don't Smoke Weed and Drive" as it is the message "Don't Drink and Drive." There is one difference, however: accidents involving marijuana are usually less fatal than alcohol-related car accidents because pot users tend to be slower drivers than drunk drivers. Still, it's very dangerous—as well as illegal—to combine either cannabis or alcohol with driving.

WARNING! POT AND PREGNANCY

Pregnant women are increasingly using marijuana for relaxation and morning sickness. (See Chapter 6.) Some epidemiological studies have found that using cannabis during pregnancy is associated with premature births, low-birth-weight babies, and miscarriages.[38] Although the data is inconclusive, given the potential risks, the American College of Obstetricians and Gynecologists,[39] the American Academy of Pediatrics,[40] and the Centers for Disease Control and Prevention[41] recommend against using pot during pregnancy and breastfeeding.

On the other hand, according to the CDC, not only have there been no reported overdose deaths from marijuana, but "fatal overdoses are unlikely."

IS MARIJUANA REALLY ADDICTING?

Unfortunately, there's no simple answer to this question, because there's no real consensus. In fact, the issue of whether marijuana is addicting is one of the most confusing and controversial cannabis topics. On the one hand, there's total consensus that marijuana can be misused and abused and is habit forming. It is, after all, a psychoactive drug. But whether marijuana is actually *addictive* is another story; it depends as much on how addiction is defined as on any objective scientific criteria.

Historically, a drug was said to be addicting if it led to tolerance—the need to increase usage to get the same results—or withdrawal symptoms, which occur when a drug user abruptly quits using the drug. Although this definition was aptly applied to heroin and other narcotics, marijuana didn't fit the bill. So marijuana was said to be nonaddicting. But that all changed in the 1970s with the War on Drugs campaign. My coauthor, Joan, had been a drug addiction researcher from the late 1960s to the early '70s. Here's Joan's take on the issue:

> *When I worked for the New York State Narcotic Addiction Control Commission and other organizations, marijuana was definitely not considered an addictive drug. Habituating, yes; but addicting, no. In 1970, the FDA declared that marijuana was a dangerous drug and designated it as a Schedule I controlled substance and federally illegal. Not long after, marijuana started being referred to as an addictive drug. This was believed to be a good strategy for preventing the increasing popularity and use of pot, especially among "hippies and lefties." The thinking was that because addiction was bad, saying marijuana was addicting would scare people off the drug.*[42] *In 1971, President Nixon started his "war on drugs," which was followed by mass incarcerations. Since then, an average of 1.5 million people a year—most of whom are Black—are arrested for possession of pot.*[43] *(See Chapter 1.) Many medical and other healthcare professionals were outraged by these dire consequences. They started to steer away from labeling and treating marijuana as an addictive drug in favor of more social and psychological approaches. So* marijuana addiction *morphed into* marijuana dependence, marijuana abuse, *and/or* marijuana-use disorder. *These terms are now generally used by healthcare professionals as a substitute for addiction. According to the most recent version of* DSM-5, *the diagnostic bible of the American Psychiatric Association:*
>
> > *[T]he word addiction is not applied as a diagnostic term in this classification. . . . The more neutral term* substance use disorder *is used to describe the wide range of the disorder, from a mild form to a severe state of chronically relapsing, compulsive drug taking. Some clinicians will choose to use* the word addiction *to describe more extreme presentations,*

> *but the word is omitted from the official DSM-5 substance use disorder diagnostic terminology because of its uncertain definition and its potentially negative connotation.*[44]

However, I still think the term *addiction* is applicable in some cases. According to the National Institute on Drug Abuse (NIDA), you can become dependent on marijuana without being addicted to it; dependence becomes addiction when someone can't stop using marijuana even though it interferes with their life.[45] NIDA admits that statistics are hard to come by, because studies don't make a distinction between dependence and addiction, but they estimate that around 9 percent of marijuana users become dependent on it. Although they don't estimate the percentage of people addicted to marijuana, it's obviously a much smaller number.

Although Joan and I might disagree on the use of the word *addiction*, regardless of what it's called—marijuana addiction, habituation, or dependence—we both believe that excessive, frequent use can be a real and potentially serious problem. This is especially true since marijuana today is much stronger than the pot Grandpa smoked. And its overuse or abuse can lead to a variety of disturbing symptoms.

Addiction to marijuana, in fact, appears to be more psychological than physiological. The good news is that actual addiction to medical marijuana is probably nonexistent since it's typically recommended that patients take some CBD along with THC, which not only decreases the risk of THC side effects, but also reduces the risk of addiction. Recently, CBD has been tapped for use as a treatment for addiction to cannabis, as well as to opioids and cocaine. Although we don't yet fully understand exactly how this works, it appears that CBD interacts with these drugs and renders them less addictive.[46]

Also, the main goal of medical marijuana use is usually relief from disturbing symptoms, not getting high. That said, as we discuss elsewhere in this book, getting high can sometimes enhance the therapeutic effects of medical marijuana or at least give patients some respite from their pain and suffering.

In any case, compared to opioid addiction, marijuana addiction is not as serious a problem.

Ironically, as we mention in Chapter 1 and describe in Chapter 4, there's increasing evidence that medical marijuana appears to actually be helping opioid addicts kick their habit.

THE M-WORD CONTROVERSY

The controversies about cannabis strains and even marijuana addiction don't hold a candle to the controversy surrounding the use of the word *marijuana* instead of *cannabis*. Both terms are often used interchangeably in both popular and professional literature. *Marijuana* is the term of choice for most consumers. *Cannabis* is not only the term preferred by the medical profession, but there is now a concerted effort by a number of cannabis experts and advocates to totally rid our dictionary of the M word! They see it as an unscientific, slangy, and stigmatized word that will make the acceptance of medical cannabis into mainstream medicine much more difficult and also dampen the chances of legalization. Anti–M worders are also concerned that marijuana has negative connotations because of its association with drug addiction and the War on Drugs.

However, just like the war against marijuana didn't stop people from using it, so the war against the word *marijuana* also seems to be a lost cause. For countless people, especially baby boomers, the word *marijuana* evokes fond memories of Woodstock, the peace movement, and flower power. Their children and grandchildren also freely use the term . . . and sometimes the drug. My coauthor, Joan, and I have had endless, sometimes heated debates about using the M word, especially in the title of this book—I against, she for. I grew up in Russia, where marijuana was and still is considered a terribly

DR. KOGAN REVISITS RUSSIA'S POT PREJUDICE

I was curious to see if Russians still held such negative viewpoints about marijuana as I did when I grew up there. To find out, I became an adviser to and coauthor of a study, which was just published, of 828 Russian medical and other healthcare students' attitudes and knowledge about medical marijuana, which is still illegal in Russia.[47] I was dismayed to find out that things hadn't changed all that much. We found that although about half the students thought medical marijuana had some significant health benefits, the overwhelming majority believed that marijuana was highly addictive and that its use posed serious physical and mental health risks.

dangerous drug. Joan, a baby boomer, had positive feelings about—and experience with—marijuana and thought I was being ridiculous. Joan won!

A recent US public opinion survey of 1,600 adults was conducted on their attitudes of the use of the M word. The researchers concluded that there was "no support for the hypothesis that calling the drug 'cannabis' as opposed to 'marijuana' will boost public support for its legalization, whether for medical use or use more generally."[48] The survey also found that people were more accepting of the use of marijuana for medical purposes rather than unspecified reasons. And many cannabis experts are now rethinking their previous opposition to the M word. According to Dr. Rachel Knox:

> *It's become more important to me that we dismantle the stigma around—and the criminalization of—the "notion" of "marijuana" than to fight what I've perceived to be an uphill battle to remove the word from legislature and the American lexicon. . . . I've also been given feedback from Mexican Americans that they feel the elimination of the word—even scientifically or medically—is another*

CANNABIS QUOTE

"Over the last two decades, the use of Marijuana/cannabis for medical purposes has become a topic of increasing interest. Scientific evidence of the safety and therapeutic potential of this ancient medicine has grown significantly to the point where its eventual rescheduling and incorporation into mainstream medical practice seems increasingly likely."

—Ilya Reznik, MD, Israeli neuropsychiatrist specializing in cannabis research[49]

affront (racially and culturally), because they use "marijuana" as medicine [so] I'm not convinced that we need to eliminate the use of the term marijuana.[50]

In fact, the terms *medical marijuana* and *medical cannabis* are frequently used interchangeably in medical journal articles and books, as well in this book. And as more states legalize marijuana, it's increasingly being recognized for its medicinal value and becoming more mainstream. So it looks like both the term—and the drug—are here to stay.

CHALLENGES TO CANNABIS RESEARCH

The bad news is that in the United States, clinical research on medical marijuana is extremely restricted and lagging behind. As my colleagues and I wrote in our recently published journal article, "There are significant barriers to research on medical marijuana, including federal policy, regulatory processes, methods of administration and standardized dosing, and standardization in research methodology."[51] But there is some hope for the future. According to a recent statement by the DEA:

The emergence of different marijuana constituents underscores the importance of research. There is a lot to learn about the impacts of marijuana and its chemical constituents. The Drug Enforcement Administration (DEA) and the Department of Justice (DOJ) fully support these research efforts, which is why a few weeks ago with the support of our interagency partners, we announced unprecedented action to further expand opportunities for scientific and medical research on marijuana in the United States.[52]

Another major obstacle is that there is currently only one DEA-approved supplier of marijuana for research purposes, which is located at the University of Mississippi and only provides marijuana to the National Institute on Drug Abuse. However, in May 2021, the DEA announced that it will soon authorize more marijuana growers who meet strict requirements to cultivate cannabis for academic researchers in the US.[53]

Unfortunately for now, the FDA refuses to approve of or even recognize that the marijuana plant can be a legitimate medicine and continues to designate cannabis as a Schedule I drug. Additionally, much of the research that is conducted uses synthetic or other pharmaceutical cannabinoids rather than the natural cannabinoids that consumers obtain through dispensaries. Also, some clinical studies combine pharmaceutical cannabinoids with medical marijuana, but review articles don't take this into account when summarizing results. So they may attribute benefits exclusively to the pharmaceutical drugs rather than giving medical cannabis the credit it's due. To confuse matters even more, most review data focuses on only a few routes of administration—primarily pills for pharmaceuticals and smoking or vaping for pot.

Because of these challenges to conducting research, both the National Academies of Sciences, Engineering, and Medicine and the American Heart Association have called for a number of changes, including funding from both private and government sources, improvements and standardization in research methodology, and relaxing FDA regulations so researchers can carry out more valid studies on short-term and long-term benefits and risks of different forms of cannabis.[54, 55] The AHA has gone even further and called for the legalization of cannabis. As they explained:

> *Because of the rapidly changing landscape of cannabis laws and marijuana use, there is a pressing need for refined policy, education of clinicians and the public, and new research . . . this should start with removal of cannabis from Schedule 1 of the US Controlled Substances Act at the federal level.*[56]

The AHA has also called for the education of the public about the different cannabis products and their active ingredients, as well as the risks of smoking and vaping, and has urged the federal government to create and require the use of standardized labeling about the THC and CBD contents in cannabis products. We discuss universal labeling in Chapter 10.

We wholeheartedly agree! But until these goals are accomplished, consumers need to educate themselves about the pros and cons of cannabis. That's why we wrote this book. We hope that this chapter has clarified the confusing cannabis terms and concepts as well as provided you with the essential information you need to make educated decisions about using medical marijuana. In the following chapters, we show how cannabis and its offshoots can help resolve many of the specific medical problems that plague us.

CHAPTER THREE

Finding the Right Route

Medical marijuana not only comes in myriad forms, but it can be taken through a variety of routes, ranging from oral to anal. Smoking pot, which has long been favored by recreational users, is also the preferred method by medical cannabis users. Vaping comes in a close second.

There are also many other effective alternatives to inhaling:

- Edibles (brownies, teas, gummies, soda, beer, etc.)
- Sublingual formulations (oils, tinctures, sprays, lozenges, etc.)
- Pills/capsules
- Topicals (creams, lotions, oils, patches, etc.)
- Rectal and vaginal suppositories

Each method has its pros and cons. The choice not only depends on individual preferences and symptoms, but also ease of use, how quickly the effects are felt, how long they last, and the possible adverse effects. Availability, convenience, and costs are other key considerations.

POT IN THE PAST

Cannabis has been administered by a variety of routes since ancient times. For example, in ancient Egypt, cannabis was inhaled, applied to the skin, put in the eyes, and inserted in the vagina and rectum.[1]

Before going into the individual routes, we'll briefly describe two important interrelated concepts that can help you understand the pros and cons of each route: bioavailability and the first-pass effect. Don't worry; they're not all that complex.

Bioavailability refers to the amount (percent) of a drug that both enters your bloodstream and is able to reach its target site. The higher the percent, the better; it means you can take a lower dose of a drug to feel its effects. Bioavailability depends on many factors, especially the route of delivery. How cannabis is consumed—smoked, vaped, swallowed, taken sublingually, applied topically, or inserted rectally—can make a big difference in its bioavailability as well as its ability to quickly bring you relief. This is where the next key concept comes in.

TABLE 3-1. ROUTES OF DELIVERY: EFFECTS AND BIOAVAILABILITY

DELIVERY ROUTE	INITIAL EFFECT	MAXIMUM EFFECT	DURATION OF EFFECT	BIOAVAILABILITY
INHALED (Smoking & Vaping)	1–3 min.	30–60 min.	2–4 hrs.	20–80%*
SUBLINGUAL	10–20 min.	30–90 min.	2–6 hrs.	15–30%
ORAL (Pills & Edibles)	60–90 min.	2–3 hrs.	4–12 hrs.	5–25%**
TOPICAL	10–30 min.	30–60 min.	1–6 hrs.	10–30%***
SUPPOSITORIES	10–30 min.	60–90 min.	2–6 hrs.	50–60%

* Bioavailability of inhaled route depends on whether smoked or vaped.

** Bioavailability of oral route depends on food consumed, other medications, weight, etc.

*** Bioavailability of topicals depends on where applied and what form (cream, patch, etc.).

The first-pass effect (aka first-pass metabolism) is a phenomenon that only affects the oral route of delivery—that is, pills and edibles. In fact, it's one of the most important factors in determining the bioavailability of oral THC and CBD. When cannabis (or any other drug) is ingested orally, it must "first pass" through the gastrointestinal system and liver where it's metabolized (broken down) before reaching the bloodstream and target tissue or organ. Hence the term *first pass*. What this means practically is that when you take THC or CBD orally, it won't kick in as quickly as when you inhale or take it sublingually. But once it does, the effects can be more potent and last longer. So you can get more bang for your buck!

INHALING: SMOKING AND VAPING

It's understandable why smoking and vaping are the favored routes of delivery; inhaling is the fastest way to feel the physical and psychoactive effects of cannabis. Both smoking and vaping avoid the first-pass effect, so the cannabis goes directly to the bloodstream. The peak levels of THC and other cannabinoids occur very quickly, usually between three and ten minutes after inhaling. And their effects usually last for an hour or two, though they can persist for up to four hours.

There are two types of vaping, and both entail heating cannabis to produce a vapor instead of smoke. The first involves vaping concentrated oil or extracts via a vape pen (aka e-pen). The second involves vaping dried cannabis flower (or buds) using a vaporizer. Although this is sometimes referred to as vaporizing, for simplicity's sake, we'll refer to the process as vaping or vaping flower. Many people prefer using a vape pen because the cannabis comes in prefilled cartridges, which they find very convenient.

However, there are some downsides. The cartridges have added chemical ingredients and may contain toxic compounds. And because they're prefilled, it may be difficult to titrate the dosages. On

POT IN THE PAST

Herodotus, the ancient Greek historian, described pot smoking in his book, *The Histories,* which was written in the fifth century BCE—2,500 years ago. And, recently, archaeologists discovered physical evidence in western China that cannabis was also smoked 2,500 years ago as part of religious rituals and for healing purposes.[2]

the other hand, vaping dry flower with a vaporizer avoids these problems; it produces potent effects while avoiding the risks of using prefilled cartridges. You can also determine how much flower to add to the vaporizer. Although vaping concentrates can deliver a high dose of THC quickly, according to a review article, "a significant proportion of medicinal users report that they prefer lower-dose forms of flower cannabis to concentrates for the very reason that effects can occur too swiftly."[3] Compared with vaping flower, vaping concentrates is more likely to lead to tolerance, which means that increasing amounts of cannabis are needed to get the same results. For these reasons, the authors conclude that vaping cannabis plant material is a better option than vaping concentrates.

Pros and Cons

There is substantial evidence that smoking and/or vaping can be effective for the relief of many symptoms, including various types of pain, sleeping problems, mood disorders, and the side effect of cancer treatment, among others. Because inhaling can deliver THC and other cannabinoids rapidly to the brain and other tissues, it can help relieve these symptoms very quickly. However, it's more difficult to get exact dosages by smoking than by vaping. And in heavy or frequent users, smoking or vaping has been linked to such respiratory problems as wheezing, chronic coughing, bronchitis, and reduced pulmonary function.[4] The good news is that there's no evidence that inhaling cannabis increases the risk of lung cancer.[5]

While both smoking and vaping can rapidly get you the relief you need, vaping is preferable for several reasons. Vaping avoids the dangers of inhaling smoke. A lower temperature is needed for vaping than smoking pot, so there's less of a chance of getting burned. Vaping also makes it easier to control dosages. That said, vaping cannabis extracts has problems of its own. The extraction process involves using artificial chemicals that can be harmful. Also, the extracts are mixed with other substances, such as oil, which has turned out to be a major problem in some cases, evidenced by the recent increase in serious respiratory illnesses and even deaths that have been linked to vaping. This new epidemic, referred to as EVALI (e-cigarette or vaping product use-associated lung injury), has affected about three thousand mostly young people in the United States and has primarily been associated with bootlegged cannabis vaping cartridges and nicotine e-cigarettes. The major culprit appears to be vitamin E acetate oil, which is illegally added to cannabis (and nicotine extract) as a thickening agent. But other additives and toxic agents may have also contributed to the problem.

Cases of EVALI have declined substantially since the peak of the epidemic in the summer of 2019. In February 2020, the CDC stopped collecting data on the disease.[6] However, it's not clear if the decline is real; there's speculation that some cases are being missed or misdiagnosed because EVALI and COVID-19 have similar symptoms.[7] In fact, California has continued to collect data and still sees occasional cases. Their department of public health continues to issue warnings about vaping: people who vape, they caution, should "avoid buying vaping products from unlicensed or informal sources, such as friends, dealers, or pop-up shops. Consumers should purchase vaping products only from licensed businesses."[8] This is sound advice no matter what state you live in! And it applies equally to all cannabis products.

Responsible members of the cannabis industry are also working to minimize the potentially harmful chemicals used in vaping devices. New technologies are allowing cannabinoids to be extracted and produced without the use of thinning or thickening agents and preservatives that may prove dangerous. Although new devices are also being developed to remove additives and contaminants and better control dosing and temperature, vaping dry flower with a vaporizer totally avoids these problems to begin with.

METHODS FOR INHALING CANNABIS[9]

METHOD OF INHALATION	TECHNIQUE	ADVANTAGES	DISADVANTAGES
Blunt	Cannabis rolled into a cigar removed of tobacco	Inexpensive, enhances effect	Harsh smoke, difficult to roll
Bong	Combusted cannabis bubbled through water	Water can trap harmful products	Expensive, less portable
Hookah	Cannabis mixed with flavored tobacco and smoke bubbled through water	Multiple users, higher volume of smoke	Combined with tobacco, potentially more pulmonary damage
Dabbing	Cannabis products chemically dissolved in solvent vapors	Easy to conceal cannabis product, potent effects	Burn injuries are common
E-pen	Cannabis concentrated into wax, oil, or hash and vaporized through e-cigarette	Discreet	Little regulation of ingredients
Joint	Cannabis rolled in paper and smoked	Convenient	Fragile and difficult to roll
Pipe	Cannabis smoked in a glass pipe	Directly inhaled, potent	Breakable, harmful resin can be inhaled
Vaporizer	Cannabis heated to below burning temperature, vapor inhaled	No smoke odor or combustion production	Expensive device, not portable, little regulation of ingredients

In addition to respiratory problems, there are other potential dangers related to inhaling. In September 2020, the American Heart Association published a review article about the negative effects of smoking and vaping on cardiovascular health (see Chapter 2).[10] And the COVID-19 pandemic has added fuel to the fire. According to a recent review article, smoking or vaping cannabis should be avoided because it can increase both the risk and severity of COVID.[11] Inhaling can also trigger coughing, which can increase the spread of the COVID virus. And sharing joints or vaping devices is definitely taboo these days.[12]

Despite these warnings, vaping and smoking pot are likely here to stay; they're the preferred delivery methods for many medical marijuana users who find them very effective for their conditions. But again, it's extremely important to weigh the risks and benefits, as well as consider the alternatives. In fact, given the risks of smoking and vaping during COVID, a recent article in *Emergency Medicine News* recommends that "patients should limit inhalation intake and switch to edibles, oils, and tinctures."[13]

SUBLINGUALS

Among all the routes of delivery, sublingual cannabis is my favorite. Putting pot under your tongue is a highly effective way to quickly get the benefits of medical marijuana without the risks of smoking or vaping. Plus, sublinguals come in a variety of forms, including tinctures, oils, sprays, and strips. Sucking cannabis-laced hard candies and lozenges is another form of sublingual delivery called "buccal." Instead of going under the tongue, they're placed inside the cheek, where they slowly melt. There are other major advantages to these tongue and cheek methods. Sublingual cannabis can be taken discreetly—no small matter if you need to take medical marijuana during work hours or even traveling across state lines, if necessary. (To be safe, be sure to keep a copy of your medical marijuana ID card with you! See Chapter 10 for more on this.)

Because sublinguals get absorbed through the mucous membranes in the mouth, they bypass the gut and liver—thus avoiding the first-pass effect mentioned above—and can rapidly enter the bloodstream. Although their effects aren't quite as quick as inhaled pot, it usually takes only between twenty and thirty minutes for sublingual cannabis to kick in. However, once it hits, the effects usually last between two and four hours, which is somewhere in between the duration of inhaled and edible routes (see Table 3-1). Because of their fairly long-lasting, continuous effects, sublinguals are ideal for many of the different conditions that we cover in this book, especially cancer and chronic neurological conditions (see Chapters 8 and 9). For example, sublinguals can be a better way to counter the gastrointestinal side effects of cancer treatment than inhaled cannabis and edibles, which can upset a patient's digestive system. On the other hand, if someone suffers from severe nausea and vomiting, putting *anything* in the mouth, including sublinguals, may be too off-putting. In that case, the inhaled route or suppositories may be a better way to go.

Because many cancer patients and those with chronic neurological conditions also take multiple medications, sublingual cannabis may be a good choice because it bypasses the gut and is thus unlikely to cause negative interactions with patients' other medications. And those patients with tremors or other physical limitations are likely to find it far easier to place cannabis under their tongues than smoking or vaping it.

As with any method, however, there are some downsides to sublinguals. Alcohol-based tinctures can be irritating and cause a burning sensation in the mouth. And some people find the distinctive taste of cannabis oil to be a real turnoff. One solution is to add olive oil or MCT oil (which is made from coconut oil) to the tincture. These oils can offset the unpleasant taste without causing mouth irritations.

CANNABINOIDS FOR CAVITIES

In addition to the sublingual, buccal, edible, and topical routes, we now have the dental route. Dental cannabinoids may be a new oral route of delivery that can get to the root of your problems, according to two recent lab studies conducted in Belgium. The researchers there discovered that CBD and other cannabinoids were more effective at reducing plaque and cavity-causing bacteria than Colgate and Oral B toothpaste and other standard dental products.[14] They also found similar results with CBD and CBG mouthwash, which worked better than mainstream mouthwash.[15]

POT PILLS

Pot pills and capsules are another convenient form in which to consume cannabis. Capsules, which are usually made from gelatin, dissolve more quickly than pills. (Since pills and capsules are basically the same, we'll refer to both as pills.) Pills are subject to the first-pass effect described above; they must first pass through the GI system and liver before reaching the bloodstream. Although it can take an hour or so for them to work, once they kick in, their effects can last quite long—up to eight hours. Pot pills may contain natural forms of THC and CBD as well as other cannabinoids and ingredients, such as terpenes—the compounds in cannabis and all other plants that give them their distinctive fragrance and flavor. These and other natural ingredients can boost effectiveness of cannabinoids, a phenomenon known as the entourage effect (see Chapter 2).

Because pot pills are flavorless, many people find them more appealing than sublinguals. Like sublinguals, their dosages are premeasured, so you know exactly what you're getting. In addition, popping a pot pill is a lot easier than smoking or vaping weed. Pills also don't require any special paraphernalia and can be discreetly carried and consumed. Plus, pills avoid the potential health risks of smoking and vaping.

However, there are also drawbacks. Some people have trouble swallowing pills. And if you take CBD pills, their bioavailability is very low; if you swallow a 25 mg CBD capsule, only about 5 mg will reach your bloodstream. While that dose can still have some benefits, you may need to take several capsules to get your desired results. Sublinguals may be a better choice because they have much higher bioavailability; you can thus take lower doses, which can save you money.

Additionally, it can take a while for the effects of pills to kick in, which can be a problem when more immediate results are needed. Also, once you swallow a pill, there's no going back. If you don't like the psychoactive or other side effects, you just have to wait it out. For many, that can be a hard pill to swallow!

EDIBLES

The edible route is, understandably, a much more popular oral delivery system than pills. In fact, eating and drinking THC- and CBD-infused food and beverages is a major craze among both recreational and medical marijuana users. And the varieties are endless: cakes, cookies, brownies, truffles, mints, caramels, teas, soda, wine, beer, and pretzels, to name but a few. Edibles that contain more than 0.3 percent THC can get you high and are federally illegal. So they can be sold only in states that have legalized medical or recreational marijuana. On the other hand, hemp-derived CBD edibles can be legally sold in stores and online. They have only trace amounts of THC, less than 0.3 percent, which is the cutoff point for determining legality—and the ability to get you high.

Edibles are an easy, tasty way to discreetly carry and consume medical marijuana. And they're a great option for anyone who has trouble swallowing capsules and/or wants to avoid vaping or smoking weed but still get the same benefits. However, THC edibles have the same effects and side effects as other forms of marijuana—including euphoria, dizziness, increased blood pressure, palpitations, cognitive impairment, and paranoia.

When marijuana is swallowed rather than inhaled, it takes the user longer—up to ninety minutes—to feel the effects. Like cannabis capsules and pills, edibles first pass through your digestive system and liver, so they're slow to reach your bloodstream and deliver their punch. And what else you eat, as well as the medications you take, can further slow things down. These and other individual factors can greatly influence the effects of edibles (and other forms of cannabis). Gender, weight, metabolism, genetics, and even previous experience with pot all come into play.

When edible effects do kick in, they can be quite long-lasting—up to twelve hours in some cases. And edibles that are high in THC can produce a very intense as well as a prolonged high. While this can be advantageous for conditions such as anxiety and sleeping problems (see Chapter 5), getting high may not be your cup of tea, especially if you have to drive or work all day. Thus, it's important to know exactly what's in an edible so you can titrate (adjust) the appropriate dose to your needs and avoid unpleasant side effects. Carefully reading the labels can be a big help.

If you're considering cannabis edibles, keep in mind that they're not all alike. THC-laced lollipops, ice pops, gum, and hard candies will hit you more quickly than cannabis cookies—as long as you don't immediately swallow the candies! As we mentioned above, these candies act as sublinguals and are absorbed through the mucous membranes in your mouth, so they go directly into your bloodstream. But while their effects may kick in more quickly, they may not last as long as those of other edibles.

CANNABIS CANDY AND KIDS

Unfortunately, cannabis-infused gummies, lollipops, and ice pops can be enticing to children, who may inadvertently eat them. While all states require childproof packaging for any cannabis-containing products, kids have been known to pry them open. The packages themselves often have appealing designs and colors that make them enticing to young kids. Tragically, there has been an increase in the number of children who overdose from edibles that were meant for adults.[16] If there are children in your home, be sure to put your edibles out of sight in a secure place where they can't see or get them.

Other Potential Problems

Edibles taste terrific, but therein lies the problem. These tasty tidbits may be just too hard to resist. And because it takes so long for edibles to take effect, it can be awfully tempting to take just one more bite or swig while waiting. To be safe, wait at least an hour or even two before indulging again. THC edibles can be especially problematic because they might give you "the munchies," which can lead to overeating or even overdosing. Indeed, an increasing number of people have wound up in the ER after overindulging in edibles. In fact, this is the top cause of healthcare visits related to cannabis intoxication and overdoses.[17] The good news is that there's no evidence that any adult has ever died from a cannabis overdose.[18]

Although cannabis-infused edibles and beverages might be helpful for some conditions—especially for those for which long-acting effects are a priority—they're rarely the best route for most medical problems. Yet while the benefits of edibles to consumers may be questionable, their benefit to the food and beverage industry is undeniable. It's predicted that annual sales of edibles will reach more than $4 billion by 2022.[19]

TOPICALS

Cannabis topicals have also delivered big bucks to the cannabis and cosmetic industries. The global CBD skin-care market alone was valued at more than $630 million in 2018 and is anticipated to reach almost $1.7 billion by 2025.[20] Cannabis and CBD topicals come in a variety of appealing forms, including creams, ointments, oils, and lip balms, among others. Not surprisingly, these products are more popular among women than men; women are more used to applying topical skin products for everything from anti-aging to zits.

Pros and Cons

While the financial benefits are clear, experts are divided over the medical benefits of cannabis topicals. Although there's increasing evidence that they can work well for pain and other problems, some believe that they don't really work and are a waste of time and money. But others (including myself) believe that topicals have an important role to play. In fact, I believe that they should be the first line of treatment for localized pain—especially muscle, joint, and back pain. Topicals can also be a superb solution for many skin disorders, including acne, eczema, and psoriasis, and even some GI problems (see Chapters 4, 6, and 7).

Unlike other routes of delivery, topicals are absorbed through the skin rather going directly to the bloodstream, the GI system, the liver, or other organs. As a result, they have fewer side effects than other routes, are safer to use with other medications, and are rarely intoxicating. And, importantly, it's virtually impossible to overdose using topicals. Although it may take some time to feel their effects, most topicals will start working within a half hour. However, with

POT IN THE PAST

Various forms of cannabis have been used topically since ancient times. For example, in ancient Egypt, cannabis was applied to wounds,[21] and in Assyria in the seventh century BC, cannabis was used topically as a bandage or an ointment to reduce swelling and bruises.[22]

joints or muscles—or other deep-target tissues—it may take an hour or so to feel their effects. The good news is that topical effects can last for quite a while—up to six hours. Allergic reactions, which may be caused by either the cannabis or whatever it's mixed with, are the most common adverse effects. To be safe, it's best to first apply the topical to a small patch of skin for two to three days to see if it causes any itching, swelling, or redness.

Some topicals contain only one specific cannabinoid, such as CBD or THC, and are referred to as "isolates." But most are whole-plant extracts, which are usually preferable. These extracts contain a variety of cannabinoids, terpenes, and other important components that work together synergistically to enhance the topical's effectiveness. This is yet another example of the entourage effect discussed

POT PATCHES

Transdermal patches have recently become quite popular; they're another very discreet and effective delivery system. Pot patches can deliver cannabis in precise dosages that can be released over many hours. This makes them ideal for muscle pain and spasms. But patches can be hard on your pocketbook. Depending on their cannabis content and concentration, some can cost as much as $15 per patch.

above and in Chapter 2. Because of the entourage effect, smaller amounts of topicals are needed to produce their therapeutic benefits, and smaller doses reduce the risk of side effects . . . and cost.

Topicals are also a prime example of another one of my favorite marijuana mantras: "Put it where it needs to go." They are not only the easiest way to do so, they're also the safest of all the routes. But suppositories come in a close second.

RECTAL AND VAGINAL SUPPOSITORIES

Last, but definitely not least, are suppositories. Rectal and vaginal suppositories are very promising methods of delivery and are another ideal way to "Put it where it needs to go." Unfortunately, many people are turned off by the idea of "putting it up the butt." But rectal suppositories can be extremely helpful for hemorrhoids, lower back and rectal or pelvic pain, and ulcerative colitis. And vaginal suppositories have a place as well. In addition to helping reduce genital and pelvic pain, there's anecdotal evidence that they can increase sexual arousal. In fact, I've had a number of patients report this added bonus to me.

Another advantage of using suppositories is that they have fewer side effects than most other routes. They bypass the gut and liver, so they have a high bioavailability rate and nearly complete absorption. What is especially interesting about suppositories is that even if they contain high doses of THC—25 to 50 mg, or even higher—many patients don't get high. This makes them especially helpful for older adults who may be prone to falls and other accidents. The only drawbacks are that they can sometimes cause diarrhea and make patients feel mildly high at doses of more than 25 mg of THC. But the biggest drawback is their high cost. In the Washington, DC, area at the present time, one pack of five suppositories of 25 mg of 1:1 CBD:THC costs $40. Because of this I often recommend that patients make their own

POT IN THE PAST

In 1889, Dr. John W. Farlow, a Boston gynecologist, published an article advocating the use of *Cannabis indica* suppositories for women's gynecological problems. He claimed that they were especially useful for women's "sensitive ovaries and in various painful affections of those organs."[23] He added that "when we take into account the usual combination of symptoms on the part of the bladder, rectum, uterus, and ovaries, and bear in mind that the suppositories can be placed directly at the seat of disease, it appears to me that there is a manifest advantage on the side of the suppositories." Farlow's sound advice is very relevant today . . . that is, if you ignore his bizarre advice for single women: "In unmarried women it is very desirable to avoid vaginal interference provided the requisite treatment can be carried out per rectum." Times have certainly changed!

suppositories. For more information on DIY suppositories, check out projectcbd.org/medicine/do-cannabis-suppositories-work.

With so many options, it's important to find the right route for you and your specific problem. The following chapters should help you do so. And, of course, no matter what route you choose, be sure to follow my favorite marijuana mantras: "Start low, go slow" and "Stop when you get to where you need to go." And if you can, "Put it where it needs to go!"

CHAPTER FOUR

Aches and Pains

Pain is the most common malady to afflict mankind and the major reason people seek medical care. And no wonder, as Will Rogers put it, "Pain is such an uncomfortable feeling that even a tiny amount of it is enough to ruin every enjoyment."[1] Chronic pain, in fact, is by far the most common reason people use medical marijuana.[2] Indeed, recent surveys estimate that more than 90 percent of medical marijuana users have used it for pain relief.[3]

There are, in fact, two types of pain: acute and chronic. Acute pain occurs suddenly, usually from an injury or disease, and is short-lived. Chronic pain, which affects 20 percent of adults in the United States (about 50 million people),[4] can severely interfere with the quality of our lives. Back pain, joint pain, nerve pain, headaches, and pain from chronic diseases all take a tremendous toll on our physical and emotional health, social and professional relationships, personal finances, and even national economics. In fact, the annual healthcare costs related to pain are over $300 billion, which is greater than the costs of heart disease, cancer, and diabetes combined.[5]

CONVENTIONAL TREATMENT FOR PAIN

The conventional treatment options for chronic pain include over-the-counter (OTC) drugs such as acetaminophen (Tylenol) and non-steroidal anti-inflammatory drugs (NSAIDs) such as aspirin, ibuprofen (Advil), and naproxen (Aleve). These over-the-counter drugs are far from safe. High doses of Tylenol (3000 mg a day or more) can cause liver damage. NSAIDs can cause kidney problems, stomach ulcers, internal bleeding, and cardiovascular problems such as high blood pressure.

Even more dangerous are opioids such as Percocet and Vicodin, which are among the most frequently prescribed, overprescribed, and misused painkillers. They're also the most addicting and dangerous prescription (Rx) drugs, as evidenced by the recent epidemic of opioid addiction, which has ruined countless lives and resulted in 49,860 opioid-related overdose deaths in the United States in 2019 alone.[6] Unfortunately, the double epidemics of opioid addiction and COVID-19 have contributed to even more recent overdose deaths; it is believed that shelter-in-place orders make it more difficult for people to seek or find addiction treatment, and in isolation, those struggling with addiction have fewer distractions to keep them from using drugs.[7]

While most opioid users don't overdose, more than 9 million Americans (twelve years and older) misused prescription opioids drugs in 2019.[8] Even when used appropriately, opioids can cause such adverse effects as constipation, dizziness, mental fog, nausea, vomiting, and breathing difficulties.

Other drugs commonly prescribed for chronic pain include antidepressants, anticonvulsives, and anti-anxiety medications. Although they're less addicting and less likely to result in overdose deaths than opioids, they have their fair share of negative side effects. Antidepressants, such as Elavil, Prozac, Zoloft, and Cymbalta, can cause dizziness, cardiac problems, nausea, constipation, and weight gain, among other adverse effects. Gabapentin (Neurontin) and other anticonvulsives that are used for nerve pain relief can cause insomnia and fatigue as well as dizziness and weight gain.

To top it all off, none of these Rx drugs are particularly effective in relieving chronic pain; they only reduce pain by about a third in most patients.[9] The good news is that there's increasing evidence that medical marijuana can fill in the pain gap.

CANNABIS TREATMENT FOR PAIN

Cannabis products have been used since ancient times for such conditions as joint pain, migraine headaches, neuropathic pain, and even convulsions, to name but a few (see Chapter 1).

And modern science backs up what our ancestors knew. The recently discovered endocannabinoid system (ECS) controls inflammation—a major source of pain—as well as pain from other causes (see Chapter 2). By activating certain receptors in the ECS, cannabis can help reduce pain and inflammation. According to a landmark report by the National Academies of Sciences, Engineering, and Medicine, "There is conclusive or substantial evidence that cannabis or cannabinoids are effective for the treatment of chronic pain in adults."[10]

CANNABIS QUOTE

"[T]he [cannabis] root eases the pains of the gout, the hard humours of knots in the joints . . . and the pains of the hips."

—*Culpeper's Complete Herbal: A Book of Natural Remedies for Ancient Ills*, 1653[11]

PHARMACEUTICAL CANNABINOIDS FOR PAIN

The FDA approved two synthetic forms of THC—Marinol (dronabinol) and Cesamet (nabilone)—which are only available by prescription, usually in pill form (see Chapters 2 and 3). Both are approved for the treatment of chemo-related nausea, and Marinol has been approved as an appetite stimulant for HIV patients but not cancer patients. Although neither of these drugs is approved for the treatment of pain, they've been studied and used for multiple sclerosis–related spasticity and pain, neuropathic pain, and other forms of chronic pain. While some studies have been encouraging, the results have been mixed. Another pharmaceutical cannabinoid, Sativex (nabiximols), is a natural, plant-derived form of cannabis that contains both THC and CBD, the nonintoxicating component of the cannabis plant. Although it's been successfully used as an oral spray in England, Canada, and other countries for MS pain and spasticity, as well as neuropathic (nerve) pain, Sativex has not yet been approved for use in the United States.

The FDA-approved pharmaceutical cannabinoids have a number of unpleasant side effects, which are similar to those of natural medical marijuana. The most common ones include dry mouth, drowsiness, dizziness, disorientation, euphoria, and feeling intoxicated.[12] Unfortunately, these drugs haven't been very effective for treating chronic pain. Nor have they been very popular with patients.

MEDICAL MARIJUANA FOR PAIN

Chronic pain sufferers generally prefer the good old-fashioned natural cannabis flower to the more modern, man-made marijuana, according to a recent review article.[13] And those who do use synthetic cannabinoids tend to quit using them because of their ineffectiveness and/or side effects. This is the result of their erratic "pharmacokinetics"—that is, how quickly they're absorbed, distributed throughout the body, metabolized, and eliminated (see Chapter 2). These factors determine a drug's effects and side effects. Compared with Rx cannabinoid pills, inhaled and some other forms of marijuana are more desirable because they work more rapidly and have fewer side effects. And, according to the review article mentioned above, "Scientific evidence indicates that the inhaled (vaporized) option is more predictable, effective, and potentially tolerable than oral preparations."[14] That said, there are some potential problems with vaping, which we discuss in Chapter 2 and later in this chapter. As with any drug, medical marijuana should be used with caution, ideally under the supervision of a physician or qualified healthcare provider.

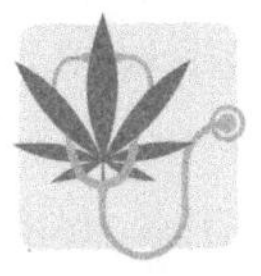

Robert, a sixty-one-year-old college professor with a history of heart attacks, had to take a high dose of statins. He started to develop severe muscle pain—a potential side effect of statins—and could no longer take long walks and jog, some of his favorite activities. He tried different statins, but the pain persisted. His cardiologist referred him to me, and I first suggested he take CoQ10—which can help to counteract statin side effects—as well as a variety of high-dose vitamins and minerals, including high-dose magnesium. Although they gave Robert some relief, the pain still interfered with his quality of life. Because it was medically important for Robert to remain on statins—and nothing else worked—I recommended that Robert apply a high concentration of THC topically. Unfortunately, it wasn't very effective, so I then recommended that he try vaping CBD along with a very low dose of THC at night. That combination worked much better. Although Robert still has some residual pain, after six months of a combination of cannabis, vitamins, and supplements, he was able to function much better and resumed his long walks and jogging.

JOINTS FOR JOINT PAIN

Joint pain is the hallmark of arthritis, a chronic condition that mostly affects women and older adults. About 27 million people in the United States have osteoarthritis, and another 1.3 million have rheumatoid arthritis, the more serious form.[15] As described above, conventional treatments are not always effective for pain and can have serious side effects, which can be especially problematic for older adults. Not surprisingly, medical marijuana is very popular among arthritis sufferers.

Although animal studies have demonstrated that smoked and other forms of cannabis can relieve joint pain, clinical studies on pot for joint pain and other problems are sorely lacking.[16] As we mention in Chapter 1 and throughout this book, because the FDA has determined that cannabis is a Schedule I drug, it's federally illegal, and therefore researchers in the United States have been thwarted in their efforts to carry out clinical research into the benefits and risks of medical marijuana.

However, according to numerous patient surveys and anecdotal evidence, not only are large numbers of patients who are suffering from joint pain turning to joints and other forms of pot for relief, most are happy with the results. For example, a recent survey of over one thousand patients in the United States with arthritis or other joint problems found that more than half had used some form of marijuana or CBD.[17] The study also found that virtually all of those who used THC (97 percent) and CBD (93 percent) said it helped reduce their pain and other symptoms. On the other hand, fewer than one in three were satisfied with their regular medical treatment.[18] The survey also looked at a subgroup of people—most of whom were suffering from rheumatoid arthritis (the most serious form of arthritis)—and found that only about 30 percent were happy with their current conventional treatment.[19] By contrast, more than 80 percent of those who used THC said their symptoms improved, and more than half substituted THC for their prescription or OTC drugs. We discuss this important "substitution effect" later in this chapter.

MARIJUANA FOR MIGRAINES

Migraine headaches are extremely painful and debilitating, and, unfortunately, extremely common. In fact, migraines are the third most common chronic illness in the United States, affecting almost 40 million people, and most sufferers are women between the ages of eighteen and forty-four.[20] As with arthritis, pot is very popular with migraine sufferers; more than one in three medical marijuana users report that headaches or migraines are their primary reason for using pot.[21] In fact, according to a large survey, almost 90 percent of people suffering from migraines or severe chronic headaches have used cannabis for their symptoms.[22] Such a high number is not surprising since many migraine patients suffer from nausea and vomiting, and cannabis has proven helpful for treating both.

There have been only a few clinical studies on the use of cannabis for migraines and other headaches, and most involve Rx pharmaceutical cannabinoids. Although these drugs hold some promise, medical marijuana does an even better job.[23] A large recent study of smoked or vaped marijuana as a treatment for migraines and other headaches found that it decreased headache and migraine pain by up to 90 percent.[24] And, according to several recent patient surveys, the majority of migraine sufferers who smoked or vaped marijuana found it to be enormously helpful, in reducing both the severity and the frequency of migraine attacks.[25]

A recent research study of migraine sufferers in Israel concluded that not only did medical cannabis reduce the long-term frequency of migraines in more than 60 percent of treated patients, but the patients also had less disability from the pain and were able to decrease their use of conventional migraine medications.[26] In fact, other patient surveys have found that the majority of marijuana-using migraine patients reduced their use of opioids and other prescription drugs by as much as 50 percent.[27]

In addition to joint pain and migraines, there's evidence that inhaled cannabis can be effective for many other painful conditions. Although most of the cannabis studies look at Rx cannabinoids instead of medical marijuana, a large review article published in 2015 in the prestigious *Journal of the American Medical Association* (*JAMA*) concluded that the "use of marijuana for chronic pain, neuropathic pain, and spasticity due to multiple sclerosis is supported by high-quality evidence."[28] More recently, others—including the National Academies of Sciences, Engineering, and Medicine—have also found evidence that smoked or inhaled cannabis can be helpful in treating some chronic painful conditions.[29] The results for Rx cannabinoids are mixed.[30]

FIBROMYALGIA

Fibromyalgia is another chronic, painful condition that mainly affects women. Approximately 10 million people in the United States suffer from this disorder,[31] which commonly causes a whole host of problems, including muscular and joint pain and stiffness, headaches, sleeping and memory problems, fatigue, depression, and anxiety. Because up to 90 percent of sufferers are women,[32] and because none of the symptoms are measurable or confirmable by tests, the medical establishment previously wrote off fibromyalgia as a psychosomatic "woman's problem." It's now finally being recognized as a "real" problem—a physical disorder of the central nervous system. Fibromyalgia is believed to be caused by a deficiency in the endocannabinoid system.[33] As described in Chapter 2, the ECS regulates all our body systems including the central nervous system. A deficiency in the system throws our bodies off-balance, which can result in low pain intolerance (a benchmark of fibromyalgia) as well as migraine headaches, sleep problems, IBS, and mood disorders. In fact, most patients with fibromyalgia (aka "fibro") tend to suffer from all these conditions.

Standard treatments for fibromyalgia are notoriously inadequate because they're either ineffective or have disturbing side effects.[34] Cannabis, on the other hand, has proven remarkedly helpful. A recent survey by the National Pain Foundation of 1,300 patients with fibromyalgia found that 30 percent (390 patients) had used marijuana. And 62 percent of those users said it was very helpful in treating their fibro symptoms.[35] By contrast, more than 60 percent reported that the FDA-approved Rx drugs for treating fibromyalgia (Cymbalta, Lyrica, and others) were not helpful at all. The National Pain Foundation concluded, "Medical marijuana is far more effective at treating symptoms of fibromyalgia than any of the three prescription drugs approved by the Food and Drug Administration to treat the disorder."[36]

It's no wonder that fibro patients are flocking to medical marijuana, especially in countries like Israel, where it's legal. A smaller Israeli survey found that 84 percent of fibro patients used pot, and more than 90 percent said they got pain relief and that their sleep improved.[37] The reason that these patients reported greater improvement than those in the US study may be because Israeli doctors tend to recommend stronger doses of inhaled THC for their pain patients. Most patients also got relief from anxiety and depression and were able to function better in their daily lives. Another study in Israel reported similar positive results, and also found that 22 percent of fibro patients who used medical marijuana quit using or reduced their dosages of opioids.[38] This is yet another example of the substitution effect (see below).

Additionally, fibromyalgia patients tend to have more complex problems that contribute to their pain, so they require more integrative approaches. For example, the main cause of their problem might actually be chronic Lyme disease, mold or heavy metals toxicities, or some other issue that is often missed by conventional practitioners. While cannabis can help, these other issues also need to be addressed.

NEUROPATHIC PAIN

Neuropathic pain, which affects about one in ten adults in the United States,[39] is the result of damage to the nervous system by injury or disease. People with this condition become overly sensitive to pain; the slightest movement or touch may cause shooting, stabbing, or burning pain. Neuropathic pain is more common in women and those over the age of fifty and most often affects the neck, lower back, and limbs.[40] It especially bothers people with diabetes and those with peripheral neuropathy, another chronic painful nerve condition that typically causes numbness, tingling, burning, muscle weakness, and sensitivity to touch and temperature, usually in the feet and legs.

Unfortunately, neuropathic pain is extremely difficult to treat. The standard treatments—opioids and other painkillers, antidepressants, and anti-epilepsy drugs—not only have potentially serious side effects, they're also ineffective for most sufferers. Cannabis, on the other hand, has shown promise in treating neuropathic pain.

There have been a number of small studies that have demonstrated the effectiveness and safety of smoked or vaped medical marijuana for treating neuropathic pain related to HIV,[41] diabetes, herpes, and traumatic injuries.[42] The authors of a 2020 review article concluded that not only was smoked marijuana effective in reducing neuropathic pain, it had very few, if any, adverse effects.[43] And, according to a large recent Canadian study, people who vaped medical marijuana for neuropathic pain for twelve months reported that their symptoms improved over the course of a year.[44]

People who have had herpes zoster (shingles) are at high risk of developing postherpetic neuralgia, another type of chronic neuropathic pain that increases with age. It's estimated that one in five people who have had shingles develop this condition, which causes severe pain in the places where the shingles rash occurred.[45] A small study in Germany found that topical cannabinoids were effective in treating the pain from postherpetic neuralgia.[46]

In addition to inhaled and topical cannabis, there's also considerable evidence that sublingual tinctures and oral sprays can reduce neuropathic pain.[47]

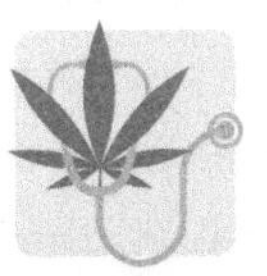

When Ellen, a high school teacher, was in her late forties, she started experiencing pain and numbness in her feet. She was diagnosed with idiopathic (unknown cause) neuropathy, which rapidly progressed. By the time she was fifty, her pain was so severe she couldn't sleep and could barely function. She became very depressed and even had suicidal thoughts. Prescription drugs (Neurontin and Cymbalta) helped to some extent, but they caused cognitive problems—including memory lapses and difficulty processing information—which made working and daily living difficult. When she came to see me, I started her on sublingual hemp-based, whole-plant (full-spectrum) CBD oil twice a day, and then added a low dose of sublingual full-spectrum THC oil at bedtime. Additionally, Ellen started an anti-inflammatory, Mediterranean-like diet and took a vitamin B complex and other supplements. After three months, most of her pain was gone and she was able to go off Neurontin and start tapering off Cymbalta. Ellen continues to take CBD and THC and is now pain-free 90 percent of the time. When she does have occasional mild flare-ups, she increases her dose of THC. She has recently switched to using a topical mixture of THC and CBD, which she applies when the pain comes back.

DR. KOGAN'S CANNABIS RECOMMENDATIONS FOR CHRONIC PAIN

When I see patients with chronic pain, I never have medical cannabis in mind as my first line of treatment. All too often, chronic pain patients haven't had the causes of their pain carefully assessed and treated. I often first refer pain patients to experts in manual medicine, including osteopathic doctors, physical therapists, and massage therapists. For countless patients, their pain is resolved, and their physical functioning is restored as a result of these referrals. Additionally, chronic pain almost always has a substantial mind/body component that hasn't been addressed before they've come to see me. Mind/body techniques, especially the widely studied mindfulness-based stress reduction programs, have been proven very helpful for chronic pain.[48]

Another very common problem I see with chronic pain is poor nutritional status and inflammation, as in Robert's case above. I estimate that at least half, if not more, of all patients with chronic pain would benefit from magnesium and B complex even if they don't have a deficiency. Once these core issues are addressed, if the pain persists, I then recommend cannabis. But the type and route of administration matter substantially.

INHALED CANNABIS

Smoking and vaping are not only the most popular methods of using recreational marijuana, they're also highly popular among medical marijuana users. A major reason is that the inhaled route works more quickly and predictably than other methods for almost all types of pain. Because inhaling works well for many of my patients, I used to commonly recommend it. But since we started writing this book, two major events occurred that have changed my mind and recommendations: the EVALI epidemic coupled with the coronavirus (COVID-19) pandemic.

As mentioned in Chapter 3, there's been an increase in serious respiratory problems requiring hospitalization, permanent lung damage, and even death from EVALI (e-cigarette or vaping product use-associated lung injury). A major culprit appears to be a common preservative, vitamin E acetate oil, but it's believed that other components may be responsible. However, EVALI primarily occurs from vaping black-market THC and some nicotine-containing e-cigarettes, and it hasn't been a problem with legitimately acquired medical marijuana vapes.[49]

While EVALI does not occur in patients who vape or smoke whole cannabis flower, the COVID risk is still a problem. Vaping or smoking cannabis during COVID can be a dangerous duet, even for young people at low risk for COVID.[50] Vaping can, in fact, increase the risk of COVID by fivefold![51] But it can be especially deadly for older adults and others at high risk. Even without these epidemics, according to a recent report by the American Heart Association, both vaping and smoking pot, like inhaling tobacco, can cause damage to the lungs, blood vessels, and heart.[52] According to the report, cannabis smoke has many of the same carcinogens and other toxins as tobacco smoke, and observational studies have linked pot smoking to heart rhythm disorders and other potentially serious cardiac problems. Although there's no evidence that smoking pot causes lung cancer, observational and other small studies have linked frequent inhaling to chronic bronchitis and other respiratory problems.

That said, if you totally understand the risks and still want to try the inhaled route, I recommend dry-flower vaping instead of smoking, which will give you a quick fix when it's needed. Vaping can also help decrease the negative effects of high-temperature smoking on the lungs. Most people need to try several strains before finding one that works well. And it's important to start with one drag, which follows one of my favorite marijuana mantras: "Start low and go slow." Because inhaled cannabis often doesn't provide lasting pain relief, you may need to take several tokes throughout the day.

EDIBLES

Although edibles are highly popular, especially among women and older adults,[53] there are hardly any studies or even surveys on whether they're actually beneficial. As we mentioned above, these studies are virtually impossible to conduct in the United States. And there are many different kinds of cannabis edibles (which includes beverages), with each product containing differing amounts of THC and/or CBD. So patients must resort to trial and error.

As we discussed in Chapter 3, edibles that contain high levels of THC may have some therapeutic value, but it can be very difficult to control the actual cannabis dose. Therefore, the effects—and side effects—are unpredictable. Also, edible effects usually take about an hour or so to kick in. On the upside, when they do, those effects can be quite long-lasting—up to twelve hours—which can be a good thing for chronic pain. So edibles (as well as cannabis capsules) can be especially helpful if you have continuous, nagging pain. And starting low and going slow is especially critical with edibles. If they're very tasty, you may be tempted to overindulge, which can lead to overdosing (see Chapter 3).

It's also reasonable for pain sufferers to experiment. For example, taking an edible containing THC at night may be the best way to get a full, pain-free night's sleep; the effects can last all night, which is not possible with inhaled weed or even sublingual forms. But if you take a THC edible in the morning, the psychoactive effects can be unpredictable, making it difficult to function during the day. In that case, there is another good option: putting it under your tongue. In my experience, patients often don't need to take any THC in the morning if their bedtime dose is high enough to fully control nighttime pain. However, sometimes the dose of THC needs to be quite high to achieve twenty-four-hour pain control. It's not uncommon for some of my patients to take 25 to 100 mg of THC at bedtime to achieve this round-the-clock effect.

SUBLINGUALS

Taking the sublingual route is usually a better choice than edibles, especially when one is just starting with cannabis, because it's more predictable. It also has many other benefits, which are described in Chapter 3.

Sublinguals are quite long-lasting, so they are ideal for many people with chronic pain. Sublingual FECO (full-extract cannabis oil) is a great way to get the effects of very high potency cannabis without smoking or vaping (see Chapter 2). FECO, which contains both THC and CBD, is one of the most commonly used and effective preparations for chronic pain and many other conditions covered in this book. My usual recommendation for patients with systemic chronic pain or pain that affects multiple areas or joints, as in rheumatoid arthritis, is to follow my marijuana mantra "Start low, go slow." I suggest a trial dose of sublingual FECO that contains 1 to 2 mg of THC, two to three times a day, and to gradually increase the dose if necessary. For most patients, between 2.5 to 10 mg does the trick. However, higher doses may be needed for some types of pain, especially fibromyalgia.

TOPICALS

Next to sublinguals, topicals come in a close second for pain. Because they can be applied at the site of pain, they're a perfect example of

SOME LIKE IT HOT

Some pain sufferers find that adding cayenne (red pepper) extract to topical cannabis is a great solution. Applying OTC capsaicin cream before or after applying topical cannabis is another good option. But be extremely careful; too much can burn your skin. And be sure to wash your hands thoroughly to avoid letting the cream touch your mucous membranes. If you do forget and touch your eyes—or, heaven help you, your genitals—you'll never do it again!

another favorite marijuana mantra: "Put it where it needs to go!" As we described in Chapter 3, topicals come in a variety of forms including creams, ointments, oils, and patches, among others.

Compared to inhaled or other forms of cannabis, it may take longer to feel the effects of topicals; however, they can last as long, if not longer, for up to six hours, so most patients find that it helps to apply them two to three times a day at the site of the pain. Cannabis patches are even better; they're time-released, so the effects can last for days. Unfortunately, patches tend to be very expensive and not all dispensaries carry them.

Recent studies have found topical cannabis to be effective for treating arthritic and neuropathic pain.[54] According to a large, recent real-time survey, the pain relief from topicals was similar to that of cannabis flower and concentrates.[55] Topicals, in fact, can act as both local analgesic and anti-inflammatory agents, so they're good alternatives to conventional pain medicines.[56] And they're far safer. As we explain in Chapter 3, the THC in topicals is absorbed through the skin rather than the lungs or stomach, so it's nonintoxicating and the side effects are rare. Outside of occasional mild allergic skin reactions, I haven't seen any adverse effects from topical use.

Many of my patients have found topicals especially helpful for muscle, joint, and some back pain. I also recommend them as the

FINDING THE RIGHT TOPICALS

Unfortunately, there aren't a lot of choices when it comes to topical products. Triple-strength topicals or very concentrated products that contain more than 500 mg of cannabinoids per jar are especially hard to find. Most dispensaries carry low-potency creams that can be very expensive once you adjust for the doses needed. If you're a DIY person, you might want to consider making your own topical preparation by adding THC or CBD tinctures to your cosmetic product. (See Appendix II: Cannabis Resources.)

first line of treatment for virtually all patients with neuropathic pain. It's definitely worth trying topicals for pain that's close to the surface, as in joint or neuropathic pain. Most of the time, I recommend that patients start with a triple topical application of 1:1:1 THC:CBD:CBDa. But I haven't seen it work well for deep back pain.

As we explained in Chapter 2, CBDa (which can be obtained from either hemp or cannabis) has similar painkilling properties as NSAIDs, such as aspirin or Motrin. In fact, milligram per milligram, CBDa is probably more effective than NSAIDs. Fortunately, a liquid form of CBDa is now fairly easy to find. But if you can't get CBDa, try a 1:1 THC:CBD cream or ointment. A number of my patients have also found that topical THCa creams can help relieve pain (see Chapter 2).

SUPPOSITORIES

Suppositories are another great way to "put it where it needs to go." Even if this makes you squirm in your seat, putting pot "up your butt" may be the best way to go! Although not nearly as popular—or appealing—as the other forms of pot, rectal and vaginal suppositories are an up-and-coming method of delivery for many conditions (see Chapter 3). Rectal suppositories can be especially helpful for pain in the lower back and rectal area, while vaginal suppositories can be helpful for women who have menstrual, genital, and pelvic pain. Indeed, vaginal suppositories were used as far back as ancient Egypt for gynecological problems.[57]

Suppositories also have a greatly reduced risk of side effects when prepared and used appropriately. They bypass the liver and have the major advantage of assuring high absorption. Plus, patients can take high doses of THC without major psychoactive effects.

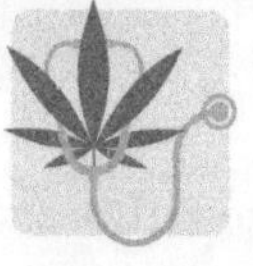

When Elana was thirty-five, she was in a terrible snowboarding accident; she hit a tree, fracturing her pelvis and rupturing her bladder. She went to every provider in the area seeking relief from her severe pelvic and bladder pain. Oral pain medications and a nerve-blocking injection didn't help at all. She also tried using a pessary and, as a last resort, underwent surgery to reposition her bladder, all to no avail. When Elana came to see me, I recommended that she use rectal cannabis suppositories vaginally. Her pain was reduced by more than half. She was thrilled! That was the first treatment that had ever had any positive effect for her. Although she wasn't completely pain-free, she was a lot more functional. I then referred Elana to a manual therapist who worked closely with her for several months. The combination of cannabis and manual therapy helped Elana return to a life without pain. As Elana pointed out, the cannabis didn't just improve her pain, but allowed her to engage more actively in physical therapy, thus speeding up her recovery.

Although there are very few studies on the use of cannabis suppositories, I find that they are one of the most effective routes of delivery for back, pelvic, vaginal, and rectal pain. I've also discovered that the use of suppositories combined with physical therapy or other manual medicine approaches often produces remarkable results for patients who have been suffering from chronic back or pelvic pain for many years. Interestingly, I've found that most manual and physical therapists who specialize in pain are much more open to cannabis as adjunct treatment than many traditional pain doctors, some of whom might still view marijuana as an addictive drug that's almost as bad as opioids.

It's also been my experience that rectal cannabis suppositories can be a godsend for older adults who have severe, inoperable back pain. Opioids and other pain medications have far too many serious side effects, which can be especially dangerous for seniors.

While suppositories aren't always perfect for pain relief, I find that they work well more often than not, especially when a patient can experiment with different doses and combinations. As with topicals, when using vaginal or rectal suppositories for pain, adding CBDa is very helpful, and I recommend 1:1:1 THC:CBD:CBDa twice daily. However, if this combination is unavailable, pure THC suppositories are very likely to work as well. In that case, I recommend starting at 2 to 5 mg of THC, and then slowly increasing the dose to as much as 50 mg. That way patients have the advantage of applying a large dose to the location of their pain. I've found that very few patients get stoned or have other side effects, even when using suppositories at a very high dose of THC.

CANNABIS COMBINATIONS

Unfortunately, there's a large gap in knowledge about which cannabinoids, combinations, and ratios might work best for different kinds of pain. Again, this is in part because there's virtually no federal funding to support this kind of clinical research. Also, Big Pharma has a vested interest in opposing this research as well as the legalization of marijuana (see Chapter 1). Fortunately, some cannabis companies are starting to step in to conduct important research on the use of cannabis and CBD on pain patients. In fact, I'm excited to be the principal investigator for one such a study, a joint collaboration between George Washington University and Cannaceutica, a private cannabis company in New York that is involved in evidence-based research on chronic pain using cannabinoid capsules. Our results should help clarify these key issues for physicians, patients, and dispensaries.

Many patients swear by the beneficial effects of CBD alone for pain, but to date, there's no clinical evidence to support this. While I've seen a number of patients who clearly have less pain after using CBD alone, the majority need at least some added THC. Our research will address this issue and answer the important question: does CBD alone work, and can it be used as a stand-alone treatment without THC in the mix?

Our joint study will be a randomized controlled clinical study, which will compare the effects of cannabis capsules containing THC and CBD versus CBD alone for patients who are suffering from chronic pain. The results should provide key information that can help physicians make evidence-based clinical decisions about the best medical cannabis treatments for their pain patients.

In the meantime, there is evidence that combining CBD with a common terpene, β-caryophyllene (BCP), can help relieve pain better than CBD alone.[58] As described in Chapter 2, terpenes not only add aroma and flavor to cannabis but can also boost its effectiveness—a phenomenon known as the entourage effect. BCP can also enhance cognition, improve digestion, and induce relaxation without sedation. While it's not easy to find hemp-derived CBD with BCP in dispensaries, some commercial websites sell it. BCP can also be found in common spices, including cinnamon, oregano, clove, and black peppercorns.

There are several lesser-known forms of THC and CBD, especially CBDa and CBG, that have been found to be effective for chronic pain and other conditions in animal studies (see Chapter 2). Unfortunately, they have rarely been studied in humans and are not yet as widely available as THC or CBD. However, increasing numbers of clinicians have reported that their patients find them helpful for some types of chronic pain.

I find that CBDa can be very helpful for inflammatory types of pain; it's now one of my standard tools for patients with inflammatory pain conditions such as rheumatoid arthritis. While some patients with these conditions may not achieve complete pain relief with CBDa, some have achieved complete or partial remission of their arthritis at high doses of 100 to 200 mg/day. I also find that CBDa combined with CBD can be especially helpful in older adults with osteoarthritis. I recommend 1:1 CBD:CBDa in an oral or sublingual dose starting at around 10 to 15 mg of CBD and CBDa twice daily, and, if needed, titrating up to as high as 50 to 100 mg of each twice daily.

I've also found that full-spectrum CBDa hemp oil in sublingual, oral, or topical form can be very effective for relieving muscle soreness from minor trauma or overexercise. In fact, I've recently seen increasing numbers of athletes who use CBD and CBDa for minor, post-exercise soreness and find it very helpful. That's a welcoming change, given that CBD and CBDa are safer in the long run than conventional medications such as Advil and Tylenol.

Adding CBG to other cannabinoids such as CBD and THC can help relieve osteoarthritis and neuropathic pain in some patients. CBG is also helpful for decreasing anxiety. However, it shouldn't be taken at night because it can be rather stimulating and may interfere with sleep. For those patients who are sensitive to any amount of THC during the day, I find that using a combination of CBD, CBDa, and CBG in the morning can be very helpful for several types of pain including neuropathic pain and inflammatory pain from osteoarthritis and other conditions. Similar to CBDa, the CBG dose is typically much lower than CBD, in the 5 to 10 mg range, taken once daily in the morning.

Finally, whatever your smallest effective dose is, that's your best dose! Be sure to follow my marijuana mantras: "Start low, go slow" and "Stop when you get to where you need to go." You'll also save money.

NEW GUIDELINES FOR CHRONIC PAIN

The Global Task Force on Dosing and Administration of Medical Cannabis in Chronic Pain convened in 2020 to develop guidelines for the use of oral cannabis for chronic pain.[59] The task force, which was made up of twenty international leaders in the field of medical cannabis, included experts in pain management, oncology, anesthesia, and psychiatry. In fall 2020, they issued a report that provides clinicians with safe and effective protocols for using medical cannabis for the treatment of chronic pain. The task force emphasized that because each patient is different, cannabis treatment—like all treatments—should be individualized. In general, however, they recommend the three approaches below. Although these guidelines refer to oral cannabis, they emphasize that "[i]f breakthrough pain management is necessary, dried flower vaporization was found to be the recommended mode of administration."[60]

ROUTINE—for treating most patients with chronic pain:

1. Start with an oral dose of 5 mg CBD-predominant cannabis twice a day. This usually means a 10:1 or so ratio of CBD:THC.
2. If needed, increase the dose by 10 mg every two or three days up to 40 mg or until the goal is reached.
3. If the 40 mg of CBD-predominant dose is inadequate, consider adding 2.5 mg of THC and slowly increase by another 2.5 mg every two to seven days to a maximum daily dose of 40 mg of THC, which can be divided into two to four administrations.

CONSERVATIVE—for elderly and frail patients—many of whom have other medical conditions and take multiple drugs:

1. Repeat steps 1 and 2 above, titrating up to a maximum dose of 40 mg a day of CBD-predominant cannabis.
2. If something stronger is needed, consider adding 1 mg of THC and adding another 1 mg every seven days until a maximum daily dose of 40 mg of THC is reached.

RAPID—meant for patients with severe pain or functional impairment and/or those who are experienced medical cannabis users:

1. Start with a 1:1 THC:CBD balanced dose of 2.5 to 5 mg once or twice a day.
2. Increase a balanced dose of THC and CBD by 2.5 to 5 mg every two or three days up to a maximum of 40 mg of THC a day.

Although these protocols were developed for clinicians, we feel they can be helpful to our readers as well. Unfortunately, most physicians and other healthcare providers—even those who are open to medical cannabis—know very little about the subject, leaving patients on their own or dependent on "budtenders" in dispensaries (see Chapter 10).

This landmark Global Task Force's report is a much-needed contribution to the effort to educate clinicians about safe and effective cannabis treatments for chronic pain. As more evidence pours in about the benefits of medical cannabis for pain relief, more physicians will be likely to recommend it to their patients not only as an effective treatment for a multitude of conditions, but as a safer substitute for opioids and other pain medications for chronic pain sufferers.

FROM GATEWAY DRUG TO EXIT DRUG

Marijuana was once demonized as a dangerous drug that leads to madness, heroin addiction, and even death! Ironically, it's now increasingly being touted as one of the best tools we have to help people cut down on, or even quit, using opioids.

Substituting cannabis for opioids is not a new concept. In 1845, the *Dispensatory of the United States* stated that cannabis was "capable of producing most of the therapeutic effects of opium, and may be employed as a substitute for that narcotic."[61] Unfortunately, it took 185 years for us to catch up. During that time, millions of lives were unnecessarily lost to addiction and imprisonment.

How did this marijuana metamorphosis materialize? Good, objective science prevailed over political proselytizing. As described in Chapter 1, it led to the discovery of the endocannabinoid system and the positive role that cannabis can play in the treatment of numerous conditions. This, in turn, has led to the legalization of medical marijuana in the majority of states.

In addition to the benefits for all the conditions described throughout this book, medical marijuana appears to be helping patients kick the very habit it was supposed to cause: opioid addiction.[62] Although more research is needed, so far it's very promising. A recent study followed 751 chronic pain sufferers who were using medical marijuana over the course of a year.[63] They not only found significant reductions in pain severity and improvement in physical and mental health, but also a significant reduction in the use of oral morphine. Their findings added to the cumulative evidence that plant-based medical marijuana is safe and effective for treating pain. The researchers concluded that marijuana is a promising substitute for opioids for treating pain as well as improving the quality of life in patients with chronic pain.

Numerous other studies and surveys of patients in states with

WARNING!

If you want to reduce your use of opioids, don't go cold turkey! Instead, taper off very gradually and *always* under the guidance of your physician. If you wean yourself off too quickly, you can experience stomach cramps, nausea, vomiting, tremors, rapid heartbeat, and high blood pressure, among other problems.

legalized marijuana find that patients significantly reduce, and in some cases totally quit, their use of opioids. In fact, studies have found that between 35 and 73 percent of pain patients in legalized states have substituted cannabis for opioids.[64] The consequences of this substitution effect are very impressive, if not mind-blowing; the states that have legalized medical marijuana have at least a 25 percent lower mortality rate from opioid overdoses than states that don't have legalized pot.[65] These studies are not only proof positive that pot is *not* a gateway drug; they provide evidence that pot can be an *exit drug*, a pathway to pain-free living.

It's expected that medical marijuana will become legal in all states in the near future. That's good news for the millions of patients suffering not just from pain but many other medical problems. The substitute effect applies to them as well. In addition to substituting cannabis for opioids, countless patients are using it in place of non-opioid prescription painkillers, benzodiazepines, antidepressants, and other potent medications. And, as you will see in the next chapters, they're finding that cannabis is a safe and effective treatment for many of their problems, including sleep disturbances, GI discomfort, skin disorders, cancer treatment side effects, and even chronic neurological conditions. Thankfully, it looks like the days of *Reefer Madness* are gone for good.

CHAPTER FIVE

Sleep and Mood

Since antiquity, marijuana has been used to treat sleep and mood disorders in countries across the globe. And for good reason. According to the authors of a recent study, "Sleep improvement, possibly alongside improvements in primary symptom management associated with sleep disturbances such as pain and anxiety, could partially explain why cannabis is the most widely used substance [of abuse] in the U.S."[1]

Sleep problems, which affect all of us at some point, occur when our sleep patterns (aka sleep architecture) are thrown out of whack. The result? Poor-quality sleep. Any number of factors, including age, health problems, diet, drugs, jet lag, job worries, and relationship problems, to name but a few, can disrupt our sleep. Traditional sleeping medications can also disrupt your sleep architecture; even if you get more hours of sleep, you may not sleep as deeply and then end up feeling drowsy all day.

Up to 70 million adults in the United States have chronic sleep-related disorders, which include insomnia, night terrors, sleep apnea, and restless leg syndrome, among others.[2] These conditions take an

SLEEP ARCHITECTURE

Sleep architecture is the term used to describe our sleep patterns because they resemble a city skyline; it refers to the four different stages of sleep. The two main types of sleep are rapid eye movement (REM) sleep, in which most of our dreams occur, and non-REM sleep, which has three different stages ranging from light to deep sleep (aka "slow-wave sleep"). REM sleep, the deepest sleep, usually occurs around ninety minutes after falling asleep. We typically cycle through all these four stages of sleep several times each night, and we usually experience longer and deeper REM sleep as morning approaches.[3]

enormous toll on sufferers and can have serious physical, emotional, and social consequences. Good sleep is restorative and essential for our well-being. Poor sleep not only profoundly affects our quality of life, it's also associated with a variety of health problems, including obesity, diabetes, hypertension, cardiovascular disease, and depression. Lack of sleep can cause problems at work, home, and school, as well as cause traffic and other accidents.

INSOMNIA

Insomnia, the most common sleep disorder, affects an estimated one-third to one-half of all adults in the United States.[4] If you're one of them, you might have trouble falling asleep, staying asleep, or both. And sleep problems may be temporary or chronic, mild or severe. While some insomnia sufferers try to tackle the problem on their own, most head to the drugstore or their doctor in search of a good night's sleep.

Conventional Treatment for Sleep Problems

Lifestyle approaches—such as cutting out caffeine, using relaxation or other mind/body techniques, and practicing good sleep hygiene (see sidebar on page 115)—are often the first line of treatment. Another non-pharmacological approach to insomnia is cognitive behavior therapy (CBT), which involves working with a therapist to change the thoughts and actions that may interfere with sleep. Indeed, CBT, which also incorporates good sleep hygiene techniques, has proven more successful than sleeping medications or other conventional treatments, and is now considered the gold standard for treating insomnia by both the American Academy of Sleep Medicine and the American College of Physicians. Unfortunately, CBT can be expensive, is not always covered by insurance, and is not available in all communities.

CBT also can help with mood disorders (see Conventional Treatments for Mood Disorders, below); in fact, sleep problems and mood are intricately connected. Poor sleep impacts our emotional as well as our physical well-being. If we don't get enough sleep, we're bound to be not only tired but irritable the next day. Chronic insomnia can have more serious effects on our mood; it can lead to anxiety and depression, making it hard to fully function in our daily lives. And when we're anxious and/or depressed, we tend to have trouble sleeping—a vicious cycle that's hard to break.

When behavioral approaches don't work, haven't been tried, or are unavailable, insomnia sufferers often turn to OTC drugs that can contain Benadryl or other antihistamines. However, these and other OTC drugs don't always work and can have disturbing side effects. Fully 80 percent of consumers who use them for insomnia experience negative effects, including drowsiness, fuzzy thinking, and memory problems, all of which can interfere with their work and social lives.[5] According to a recent study, long-term use of Benadryl could increase the risk of dementia.[6] However, many herbal or other natural supplements—including melatonin, magnesium, tryptophan, valerian root, lavender extract, lemon balm, and chamomile tea—have been found to be helpful in promoting sleep and are often safer than OTC and prescription drugs when used at recommended dosages.

If OTC drugs or supplements don't do the trick—or the side effects are too unpleasant—insomnia sufferers are often prescribed sedatives or hypnotics, such as Ambien and Lunesta, or benzodiazepines, including Valium, Xanax, and Klonopin. An estimated 8.5 million adults in the United States use these drugs.[7] However, they haven't been FDA approved for chronic insomnia and shouldn't be used for more than a few weeks. Prescription sleeping pills have been linked to memory loss, sleepwalking, falls, and other accidents, and even suicide.[8] Benzodiazepines, which are also used for anxiety and depression, are responsible for almost 12,000 overdose deaths a year.[9] A recent study of more than 10,500 patients who were prescribed hypnotics found that they were at a significantly increased risk of dying or developing cancer within the following two and a half years.[10]

In addition to the risks of Rx and OTC sleep medications, approximately half of the people who use them are dissatisfied with the results.[11] It's no wonder that so many insomnia sufferers are turning to medical marijuana in hopes of getting some shut-eye. And for many, their dreams are coming true.

POT IN THE PAST

"The Indian hemp is, among the known anaesthetic drugs, the narcosis which most perfectly achieves a replacement of natural sleep . . . without bad repercussions."

—German researcher Bernard Fronmueller, 1869[12]

Cannabis Treatment for Sleep Problems

As we explained in Chapter 3, the endocannabinoid system (ECS) helps regulate our major body functions, including sleep. More specifically, the ECS controls our circadian sleep–wake cycles and helps promote and maintain sleep.[13] Cannabis can activate the ECS receptors and affect our circadian rhythms and our sleep–wake cycles.[14] Therefore, according to a major report on the health effects of cannabis by the National Academies of Sciences, Engineering, and Medicine, "cannabinoids could have a role in treating sleep disorders."[15]

It has only been since the 1970s that studies about the effects of cannabis on sleep patterns have been conducted. Most have been lab studies involving rats and mice, and the results have been mixed. More recently, however, there have been a number of small studies involving real people instead of rodents. They focused on the effects of cannabis on sleep patterns rather than on insomnia and also had mixed results, according to a comprehensive review of human and animal studies.[16] This is not surprising since most of these human studies tended to be poorly designed, and some involved very few subjects. These studies also involved pharmaceutical cannabinoids (nabilone and dronabinol) rather than natural, plant-based THC and/or CBD. Despite these drawbacks, the review article concluded that using cannabis, at least for the short term, appears to be effective in helping people fall and stay asleep and have deeper, more restorative sleep.[17]

The article also concluded that the dosage and type of cannabis makes a difference. There is conflicting information on whether a higher dose of THC or CBD works better; some studies found high-dose THC had a sedating effect, while low-dose CBD tended to have a stimulating effect and has been associated with increased wakefulness. By contrast, other studies found that a high dose of CBD had a sedating effect and helped subjects sleep longer hours with less interruption. The authors of the review article concluded that patients might benefit from combining a high dose of CBD with a low dose of THC.

However, in my clinical practice, I have found that the effects of THC and CBD on sleep are variable. Most of my patients report that THC is more beneficial for sleep than other cannabinoids; some claim that high doses of CBD work very well for them. More clinical studies are needed to clarify what forms of cannabis are best for sleep.

The good news is that there have been some recent large-scale surveys of people who use plant-based cannabis for insomnia. For example, a survey of more than 1,500 medical marijuana users found that about two-thirds of those with sleep problems decreased their use of sleeping medications.[18] This is another example of the substitution effect, a phenomenon in which patients substitute cannabis for their pain or other medications (see Chapter 4).

Another study of more than 400 insomnia sufferers who smoked or vaped cannabis flower found that the majority experienced a significant improvement in their sleep.[19] *Cannabis indica* users also had more symptom relief and fewer side effects than those who used *Cannabis sativa*. The delivery route was also key; people who vaped or smoked pipes had more symptom relief than those who smoked joints.

As we mentioned in Chapter 2, cannabis experts claim that there is no real distinction between *sativa* and *indica*. The effects of each depend on the other contents, especially terpenes for sleep disorders. Rather than focusing on *sativa*, *indica*, or hybrids, look for strains that contain myrcene, linalool, and β-caryophyllene, which are especially helpful for pain-related sleep problems.

Unfortunately, studies are lacking on sublingual tinctures and edibles for sleeping problems. Still, it's clear that cannabis is not only helpful for treating insomnia, it's a safer alternative to and usually more effective than both prescription and OTC drugs. Despite the lack of studies, sublinguals and edibles may make the most sense for patients who have a hard time staying asleep, because their effects last much longer than inhaled weed (see Chapter 2). So having milk and a cannabis cookie at bedtime is better than smoking a joint.

As mentioned above, many people substitute cannabis for sleeping and pain medications. Indeed, pain and sleep are intricately connected. In fact, nighttime pain is one of the major causes of insomnia. It's a vicious cycle: the more pain, the less sleep. The less sleep, the more pain. A recent large-scale survey determined that sleep problems and pain were the major reasons people used medical marijuana, and most found it helpful for both problems.[20] So even if pain (or pleasure, for that matter) is the major reason someone uses weed, they're likely to reap the additional bonus of having a better night's sleep!

Dr. Kogan's Cannabis Recommendations for Sleep Problems

Out of all the symptoms I see in my practice, sleep problems are among the most important; they affect every aspect of a patient's life. If someone doesn't sleep well, all their other problems will worsen. So sleep is often the first symptom that I concentrate on, not only because it's usually the easiest one to improve, but because other conditions are difficult to treat if someone is not sleeping well.

Dispensaries often recommend pure THC products for sleep problems. However, combining THC with CBD decreases the chances of side effects, so I usually start patients with a low dose of a combination of sublingual THC and CBD. Speaking of side effects, most potentially disturbing cannabis-related side effects go away while you sleep. But if there are any morning side effects, they tend to be fewer and less intense compared with conventional sleeping medications.

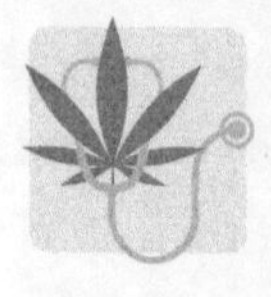

Sarah, a sixty-five-year-old business executive, was at her wits' end. She had been suffering from severe insomnia for more than twenty years and was now

sleeping only three to five hours a night. As a result, Sarah could barely function mentally and physically. The Ambien she was given at a sleep center helped her fall asleep, but she still complained that she felt tired and couldn't think clearly during the day. Although she loved her job, she decided she had to retire. When I first saw her, I recommended that she initially try integrative approaches, including yoga, acupressure, herbs, and biofeedback. While somewhat helpful, they didn't really change her sleep patterns enough to improve her quality of life. I decided that a more aggressive approach was needed and started her on a sublingual sleep tincture of a mixture of CBD and THC. Within a month, Sarah felt so much better that she tapered down her Ambien and started sleeping seven to eight hours a night. She told me that she was now feeling more energy than she did in her fifties and was considering going back to work. At a recent follow-up, Sarah told me she still uses her sleep tincture on a somewhat regular basis and has not taken Ambien for years.

My patients who have the hardest time falling asleep often have the best responses; they tend to respond quickly—usually within a few days. They have said things like, "Oh, my God, where were you before? I slept better right after the first dose." Even if it takes longer for the pot to kick in, most are very pleased with the results.

If you have difficulty falling asleep, try a sublingual tincture of 3 to 10 mg of 1:1 THC:CBD. If you haven't had THC before, start out with a very small amount: 1 mg at the most. It's important that whatever product you choose should contain calming terpenes, such as myrcene or linalool (see Chapter 2). In many dispensaries patients can find sublingual FECO (full-extract cannabis oil) or alcohol tinctures of THC combined with an equal amount of CBN (cannabinol), which my patients say works really well. As described in Chapter 2, CBN is a mildly psychoactive, nonintoxicating cannabinoid that is usually present in small amounts in cannabis.

Whatever you use, take it an hour before bedtime for three days. If you need more, increase the dose by 1 mg of THC each night until you get the response you need. As soon as you find an effective dose, *do not* increase it any further. It will not be more effective, and you may experience more side effects, which can include dizziness and morning drowsiness. So be sure to follow my marijuana mantras: "Start low, go slow" and "Stop when you get to where you need to go."

If you don't have trouble falling asleep but wake up in the middle of the night and can't fall back asleep, I recommend 1:1 THC:CBD by the oral route, either as capsules or edibles. When you take cannabis orally, it takes longer to get absorbed, so the effects take longer to kick in. This is because it first passes through the GI system and liver before reaching the bloodstream, referred to as the "first-pass effect" (see Chapter 3). Although you'll have a delayed reaction, the effects will last longer. But they may also be more intense. If you prefer to smoke or vape, consider combining it with sublingual or edible cannabis because it's hard to get an exact dose by just inhaling. And because the effects of inhaled weed don't last very long, the addition of oral cannabis can keep you asleep longer.

There's some concern that people who use cannabis for a long time may develop tolerance and need to increase their dose to get the same sleep benefits,[21] which is the case with a few of my patients. However, some researchers believe that tolerance doesn't occur when using low doses, that the body gets used to better sleep and continues doing well after using cannabis for a period of time on a low dosage, and that patients are very unlikely to develop tolerance with cautious, intermittent use. I have a lot of patients who come back after a couple of months and say, "I don't feel I have to use as much. I just keep it by my bedside to use occasionally when I'm stressed and can't fall asleep." In fact, most tell me that once their sleep improves, they only use it intermittently when their needs change with increased stressors, life transitions, travel, or other life disruptions. But by then they know what dosage works best and can easily regulate their weed and sleep. It's the opposite of tolerance! And a number of my patients totally stop using it. Cannabis, in fact, can be curative for some people with sleeping problems.

I'm often asked by patients if taking CBD at bedtime would help them sleep. I find that while it sometimes can help, the doses often need to be quite high—more than 100 mg—to work, I commonly find that those patients who swear that CBD works for their insomnia are the ones whose insomnia is driven by anxiety. For them, CBD can be a great tool. They should start with 15 to 30 mg a few hours before bedtime and titrate up by 15 to 20 mg every night until they find a minimally effective dose.

For those people with severe chronic sleep problems who may need to keep taking cannabis regularly, their best solution is to learn *why* they're not sleeping. For them, psychotherapy, cognitive behavioral therapy, and lifestyle changes can be especially helpful. In fact, as

GOOD SLEEP HYGIENE

- Go to bed at the same time every night and wake up at the same time every morning.
- Keep your bedroom dark, quiet, and cool (under 68 degrees).
- Avoid checking your clock at night.
- Avoid large meals, caffeine, nicotine, and alcohol before bedtime.
- Avoid or limit naps to twenty to thirty minutes.
- Avoid strenuous exercise four to six hours before bedtime, but get some exercise each day.
- Relax before bedtime: try a warm bath, soothing music, a massage, or anything else that relaxes your mind and body.
- Avoid watching political or other potentially disturbing programs.
- Don't talk to or text with annoying people before bedtime.
- And last but not least—TURN OFF YOUR CELL PHONE AND PUT IT IN ANOTHER ROOM!

good as medical cannabis is for insomnia, anyone suffering from sleeping problems should practice good sleep hygiene.

The one insomnia mantra that you constantly hear from all sleep specialists is "Bed is only for sleep and sex." But this mantra tends to be ignored by people who love to read or watch TV in bed. On the other hand, others may find this great advice, especially when pot is part of the picture. In fact, pot, sex, and sleep can make a terrific threesome, as many of my patients have happily discovered.

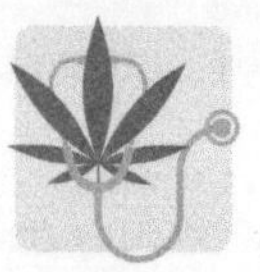

Barbara was in her mid-seventies and suffering from serious insomnia. Mindfulness, supplements, and even Valium didn't help, so I recommended a low-dose sublingual tincture of 1:1 THC:CBD. She recently sent me the following note: "Thanks to your wise guidance and a tincture of THC:CBD, this chronic insomniac can now fall asleep—and sleep through the night—without pharmaceuticals. And I feel clearheaded and energized the following morning. AND, also thanks to the THC, my husband and I can have terrific sex practically every night."

Marijuana has long been considered an aphrodisiac (something that makes you feel sexy), as well as a soporific (something that makes you sleepy)! And stoned sex is not just for twenty-year-olds;

POT IN THE PAST

"If the resin be swallowed, almost invariably the inebriation is of the most cheerful kind, causing the person to sing and dance, to eat food with great relish, and to seek aphrodisiac enjoyment. The intoxication lasts about three hours, when sleep supervenes."

—W. Ley, "Observations on the Cannabis Indica, or Indian Hemp," 1843[22]

---

it's even better for older people. So *my* mantra is "Bed is only for sleep and sex . . . and occasionally pot." However, my advice about having stoned sex is certainly not set in stone! It's clearly a very personal matter. But if you do go for it, don't overdo it: one study on the impact of marijuana on the libido found that "a small amount of cannabis tends to energize, while a large amount can be sedating."[23] So when it comes to cannabis and sexual pleasure, a little less weed might mean a lot more fun. Plus, using THC-containing lubricants can be a great way to enhance your and your partner's mutual pleasure.

NIGHT TERRORS AND POST-TRAUMATIC STRESS DISORDER (PTSD)

Not only is medical cannabis a godsend to the sleep deprived, there's increasing evidence that it can help people suffering from what is arguably the most disturbing and debilitating sleep disorders: recurrent night terrors or nightmares. These conditions are, unfortunately, very common in adults suffering from post-traumatic stress disorder, which affects about 8 million adults in the United States.[24] Indeed, recurrent

COMMON PTSD SYMPTOMS

In addition to night terrors, other symptoms of PTSD include:

- Psychological problems: vivid flashbacks, fear, mistrust, and severe anxiety.
- Behavioral problems: agitation, irritability, hostility, hypervigilance, self-destructive behavior, or social isolation.
- Emotional/mood problems: loss of interest or pleasure in activities, guilt, loneliness, emotional detachment, unwanted thoughts, and angry outbursts.

nightmares are considered to be the hallmark of PTSD, affecting an estimated 71 to 96 percent of people with this condition.[25]

Although PTSD disproportionately affects military veterans, many victims of sexual or physical abuse, violent crimes, terrorist attacks, and serious accidents, among others, also suffer from PTSD.

Whatever the cause, their nightmares often involve reenactments of the initial trauma and are accompanied by intense fear and anxiety—sometimes involving screaming and physically acting out the traumatic event. Falling back asleep after such episodes becomes exceedingly difficult, if not impossible.

Conventional Treatment for Night Terrors and PTSD

Conventional treatments for night terrors and PTSD typically involve Rx drugs—such as sedatives, antidepressants, antipsychotics, and anticonvulsives—and/or psychotherapy, CBT, or other behavioral approaches. While these therapies, especially CBT, have proven helpful,[26] most medications have not. Plus, they all have potentially serious side effects.[27]

Cannabis for Night Terrors and PTSD

Veterans suffering from PTSD have been self-medicating with marijuana for decades to help cope with the often-debilitating symptoms. And they're onto something. Although some veterans may abuse drugs, including marijuana, there's growing evidence that cannabis can be effective not only for treating night terrors but for many of the other symptoms of PTSD.[28] Medical marijuana has been shown to reduce the frequency of nightmares, and the combination of THC and CBD appears to be especially helpful for treating both PTSD-related night terrors and insomnia.[29]

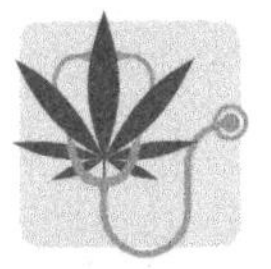

David, seventy, had been suffering from frightening night terrors for decades. He would awaken several times each night filled with anxiety, shaking, and covered in sweat. None of the doctors he consulted could help. He decided he would try anything and go anywhere to find a cure and wound up traveling to both the Cleveland and Mayo Clinics. Their treatments were similar: lifestyle adjustments, sleeping pills, antidepressants, anti-anxiety pills, and high dosages of antipsychotics. Although some of these drugs helped him sleep through the night, none were able to rid him of the night terrors. The Mayo Clinic even recommended that he try shock therapy, which he refused. When he returned home, he found a new sleep specialist and asked him about medical marijuana, which David had just read could help with sleep disorders. The doctor referred him to me; I recommended that he take a sleep tincture that was a combination of THC and CBD. After the first dose, David called me and said, "I don't know what it is, but it's a miracle. I slept through the whole night and all my night terrors were gone!"

CANNABIS CATCH-22

Due to a "cannabis catch-22," veterans suffering from PTSD can't get marijuana at VA hospitals or from VA doctors. The U.S. Department of Veterans Affairs is run by the federal government, and cannabis is federally illegal. But there is some hope for veterans—and all Americans. In 2019, the House Committee on Veterans Affairs passed two bills: one would allow researchers to conduct clinical trials on the effects of marijuana on PTSD, chronic pain, and other problems that typically affect veterans; and the second would allow VA doctors to recommend medical marijuana to their patients. But don't get your hopes too high—there's still a catch. To take effect, the bills have to pass both the House and the Senate, and finally be signed into law by the president.[30]

In fact, PTSD is one of the approved conditions for using marijuana in many of the states where medical cannabis is legal. It is also one of the most common reasons some veterans' groups have been pushing for legalization and allowing VA doctors to recommend it for their patients.

Dr. Kogan's Cannabis Recommendations for Night Terrors and PTSD

My recommendations for night terrors are virtually the same as for any sleep problems. Because I'm a general internist, I've had rather limited experience specifically treating PTSD. That said, I have worked closely with veterans for several years while helping to set up the VA Integrative Health and Wellness Program in DC. What I have heard from my colleagues or read is that most people with PTSD who use medical cannabis find that smoking or vaping weed that's high in THC can help control their symptoms. And the side effects of high doses of THC, especially increased anxiety, can be minimized by adding CBD.

Integrative Approaches for Night Terrors and PTSD

While weed can do wonders for sleep disorders and PTSD, other integrative approaches can also be remarkably effective.

These include:

- Acupuncture
- Meditation
- Hypnosis
- Yoga
- Biofeedback
- Herbs and essential oils
- CBT and other forms of therapy

These approaches can also be extremely helpful for mood problems, especially anxiety and depression, either with or without medical marijuana.

MOOD PROBLEMS

Most of us experience mood problems at various times during our lives. What keeps us up at night can also make us feel anxious or depressed during the day. The biggest culprits—family finances, work, politics, and health—are now even more troublesome thanks to the COVID-19 pandemic. Increasing numbers of people are thus turning to marijuana for relaxation and relief from isolation, anxiety, and depression, as evidenced by the huge spike in retail sales.[31] Not only have sales of pot increased, most states that have legalized marijuana have declared dispensaries an essential service.

Although some of the increase in sales may be to new customers, those who already use marijuana for medical reasons have also increased their consumption dramatically. According to a recent survey of more than 1,200 medical marijuana users, 38 percent have consumed more pot since the start of the pandemic. And those who were suffering from anxiety and depression increased their use by a whopping 91 percent![32]

Cannabis has been consumed for centuries to help reduce stress and relieve anxiety and enhance mood. In fact, these are among the top reasons people use both medical and recreational marijuana.[33] According to numerous review articles, surveys, small studies, and anecdotal evidence, marijuana users are not only happy with the results, many are substituting cannabis for conventional treatment.[34] This substitution effect is discussed in Chapter 4. While many people are turning to medical marijuana for their mood problems, most first seek conventional treatments from their primary care physicians, psychiatrists, or other mental health professionals.

Conventional Treatment for Mood Problems

Seeking relief from anxiety and depression are among the top reasons people go to doctors.[35] Depending on whom they go to, they may receive psychological solutions or pharmaceutical ones. CBT is considered the treatment of choice for anxiety[36] as well as the safest for both anxiety and sleeping disorders. If CBT or psychotherapy are unavailable, unaffordable, or unacceptable, patients are likely to see a physician who will prescribe antianxiety and anti-depression medications.

Many of those who use marijuana for mood problems have previously tried these conventional drug treatments and have been dissatisfied with the results or are concerned about the side effects. These drugs are often the same ones prescribed for sleeping problems and have the same potentially serious side effects mentioned above. Selective serotonin reuptake inhibitors (SSRIs)—such as Prozac and Zoloft—are also commonly used to treat anxiety and depression but can cause drowsiness, weight gain, and sexual problems, among others.

Cannabis Treatment for Mood Problems

For the past one hundred years, marijuana has been viewed as a dangerous drug that can cause mental illness . . . or worse. This *Reefer Madness* mentality still persists, and marijuana is still stigmatized by many patients and physicians alike. Because of this prejudice against pot—and the federal laws that have prohibited or severely limited its use in clinical studies—the therapeutic benefits of cannabis on mood in healthy adults is a subject that has largely been ignored by researchers.

Unfortunately, the clinical research and surveys that have been conducted tend to focus on the health hazards rather than the health benefits of marijuana. And these studies often involve illegal, recreational marijuana use and abuse, especially by adolescents. In addition, many of the subjects are chronic marijuana and multidrug users who have serious mental health problems, such as bipolar disorder and schizophrenia. Not surprisingly, most of these studies have found that cannabis is associated with mental health problems. But this finding is now being refuted. According to the National Academies of Sciences, Engineering, and Medicine report mentioned above, although there is evidence that heavy cannabis use in some people may contribute to psychiatric disorders, in general, cannabis doesn't appear to increase anxiety and depressive disorders.[37]

There have been some clinical marijuana mood studies, but they typically involved Rx pharmaceutical cannabinoids. So their results—which are often mixed—may not apply to the use of natural, plant-based cannabis. In general, however, there is consensus that cannabis can either be *anxiogenic* (cause anxiety) or *anxiolytic* (calm anxiety), depending on the THC:CBD ratio, dosage, and terpenes. For example, high doses of THC (more than 10 mg) have been shown to cause anxiety, panic, and paranoia in healthy adults, while low doses of THC (less than 2 mg) has been shown to help reduce anxiety and depression in healthy people, as well as in those suffering from cancer and other chronic diseases.[38] However, compared to THC, the anti-anxiety effects of CBD are much more consistent and reliable. Not only can CBD effectively reduce anxiety, it can also counteract the

---

WARNING!

THC has been known to precipitate psychological problems or even psychosis in some people, especially adolescents who are heavy users and people with a history of psychiatric disorders. So if you are currently experiencing severe anxiety or depression, or have in the past, be sure to consult a psychiatrist or other mental health professional before using any form of cannabis for any reason.

---

anxiety-causing effects of THC.[39] In fact, the combination of THC and CBD has been found to be especially effective in reducing anxiety.[40] Additionally—and possibly even more important—is the terpenes content. The presence of calming terpenes such as myrcene, β-caryophyllene, and linalool can increase or balance the effects of THC and CBD.

The positive effects of cannabis on anxiety are further confirmed by the substitution effect discussed above. Numerous online and dispensary surveys of patients find that while large numbers of them are substituting pot for their prescription opioids, many others are replacing their anti-anxiety or antidepressant meds with cannabis.[41] This high substitution rate is further support that cannabis may be an effective treatment for mood disorders.[42]

Two large studies were recently published that specifically looked at the effect of inhaled cannabis on mood. The first was a Canadian study of 1,399 medical marijuana users who retrospectively reported their symptoms of depression, anxiety, and stress on a mobile app.[43] The study found that shortly after use, cannabis significantly reduced the subjects' ratings of depression, anxiety, and stress. Interestingly, women experienced greater reductions in anxiety than men. The study also found that cannabis that was low in THC and high in CBD was more helpful for depression, while a high THC/high CBD combination was better for stress reduction. The effects, however, appeared to be temporary; long-term use of cannabis didn't result in further reduction of mood problems and, in some cases, made them worse.

The second—an American study that involved a similar mobile app—examined in real time how inhaling cannabis flower affected depression in 1,819 people.[44] The researchers reported that more than 95 percent of their patients experienced relief from depression, most within two hours or less of inhaling. They also found that there were minimal, if any, adverse effects. According to the authors, given these results, "it is understandable why some patients might choose to replace or augment their conventional pharmaceutical antidepres-

POT IN THE PAST

"I have no hesitation in affirming that in my hands [Cannabis sativa] has usually, and with remarkably few substantial exceptions, been followed by manifest effects as a soporific or hypnotic in conciliating sleep . . . and as a nervine stimulant in removing languor and anxiety, and raising the pulse and spirits; and that these effects have been observed in both acute and chronic affections, in young and old, male and female."

—John Clendinning, "Observations on the Medicinal Properties of the Cannabis Sativa of India," 1843[45]

sant treatment with medical Cannabis when given the legal opportunity to do so. Our results indicate that THC in particular is positively correlated with an immediate reduction in the intensity of depressive feelings."[46]

Dr. Kogan's Cannabis Recommendations for Mood Problems

Depression

Depression is very strongly associated with sleep disturbances; when sleep gets better, depression often improves. So addressing any sleep problems with good sleep hygiene and other integrative approaches is a good place to start. Even if sleep isn't a problem, the various integrative methods mentioned above should definitely be tried before using medical cannabis.

However, if they fail, taking a low dose of THC (0.5 to 2 mg) twice a day sublingually can often do the trick. Sublingual energizing FECO that contains uplifting terpenes, such as pinene and β-caryophyllene, can be particularly helpful for depression-related cognitive fatigue and brain fog. Oral THC (capsules or edibles) can also be a good choice if a small dose is needed. While the longer-lasting effects from oral cannabis can be a plus, the sublingual route is preferable; its effects are more predictable and are not diluted by food.

Many of my patients who have a long history of using cannabis prefer to vape or smoke pot for their depression. Although the inhaled route is usually not my first choice because of the possibility of respiratory side effects, switching to other forms is not always easy. Chapter 3 explains the pros and cons of the various routes of administration.

My most recent tool for helping patients with depression is CBG. Like CBD, CBG can be derived from hemp and is therefore legal (see Chapter 2). However, in contrast to CBD, which primarily has anti-anxiety effects, CBG can have significant mood-enhancing and energizing effects. In fact, some of my patients report that it is so energizing, that they can't take it past noon because it disrupts their sleep. CBG can also be combined with all other cannabis regimens. I suggest taking it in the morning at a starting dose of around 3 to 5 mg. Although most patients ultimately need between 10 and 25 mg, some patients respond well to lower doses.

Anxiety

Because anxiety often responds well to moderate doses of CBD, that's frequently a good place to start. I usually recommend beginning with 10 to 15 mg of sublingual CBD oil twice a day, which works for most people. (For older people, the initial dose could be as low as 5 mg.) If that dose doesn't help, it can be titrated up to as much as 75 mg twice daily. While sublingual forms of CBD are clearly the best option, vaping dry flower or oil high in CBD can also be very effective. However, if sublingual CBD is used, high doses (i.e., several hundred milligrams) are rarely needed for most patients.

Another important advantage to using CBD is that it's usually hemp-derived, and therefore legal and widely available in most states (see Chapter 2). Just make sure you get high-quality products from a reputable company, given the fact that the market is largely unregulated.

If the CBD doesn't do the trick and you decide to use THC-containing products, try a very low dose of 0.5 to 2 mg of THC twice daily. Such microdosing can be quite effective. If higher doses are needed, gradually titrate up until you find a dose that works, then stop increasing the dose, thus following my marijuana mantras: "Start low, go slow" and "Stop when you get to where you need to go!"

Since CBD is often effective for anxiety, products with a high CBD to THC ratio are usually the best bet when pure CBD doesn't work—10:1 or even 20:1 CBD:THC products are available in most dispensaries. Some people prefer to take CBD and THC separately at different times of the day. This is because THC-containing products can cause psychoactive effects, which may interfere with work and other daily activities. But these effects can also be very helpful for mood problems. Several of my patients have described that after the initial high, THC had strong antidepressant and anti-anxiety effects.

Keep in mind that sleep issues and emotional problems are highly subjective and hard to measure. So the best product, dose, and even route can vary with each person. What I have found is that most patients experiment on their own until they find the best mix or best strains for anxiety, sleep, and depression. Many of my patients eventually end up taking several different forms and dosages of cannabis. For patients who have a combination of pain, depression, and insomnia (a very common trio!), I recommend a 1:1 THC:CBD sublingual sleep tincture at bedtime, and a tincture or vape of stimulating THC-containing strains during the day to control pain and depression. I also sometimes recommend extra CBD to minimize THC's psychoactive effects.

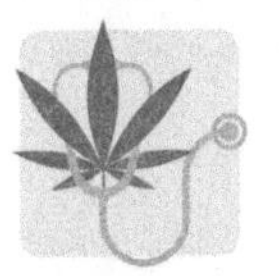

When Carol, a seventy-eight-year-old retired accountant, came to see me, she was desperate for relief; her chronic depression, anxiety, insomnia, and back pain were causing her immense suffering. She had also lost fifteen pounds and now weighed under one hundred pounds. She felt so

miserable, she had even considered taking her own life. Antidepressants didn't work well and sleeping medications caused terrible side effects, including morning lethargy and brain fog that interfered with her daily routine. She also took an opioid (oxycodone) for pain. Carol had been in psychotherapy for many years, which she said hadn't helped her that much. I started her on 1:1 THC:CBD sublingual drops at bedtime combined with 10:1 CBD:THC topical cream for the pain. In addition, I recommended high CBD:THC ratio sublingual drops in the morning for her anxiety.

When I saw Carol for her three-month follow-up, she was doing extremely well with the medical cannabis. She had stopped taking all her prescription medications except an occasional low dose of oxycodone when her back pain flared up. Interestingly, she found psychotherapy to be much more helpful once she started using cannabis. At her most recent follow-up she told me, "This pot has changed my life! I'm relaxed, less depressed, and can sleep! You can't imagine how much better my body feels with these changes! My quality of life is so much better now." Carol's encouraging report was confirmed with a modest but clear ten-pound weight gain and, what is probably most significant, she was able to function much better and feel positive about her life.

As helpful as medical cannabis can be in some cases, finding and addressing the root cause of the chronic depression, anxiety, and severe insomnia is even more important. The best long-term treatment plan for such problems typically involves some form of psychotherapy or counseling. That said, given the key role that the ECS plays in sleep and emotions, medical marijuana can play a major role in treating these problems.

CHAPTER SIX

Gastrointestinal Disorders

Some of our most common, sometimes gut-wrenching, and often embarrassing problems are related to our stomach, digestion, and bowels. And more and more people are finding that medical marijuana gives them relief from their gastrointestinal (GI) disorders, such as gastroesophageal reflux disease (GERD), irritable bowel syndrome (IBS), and inflammatory bowel disease (IBD). In fact, cannabis has been used to treat many of these and other GI problems for centuries, and there's now increasing evidence that it does indeed work.

POT IN THE PAST

In India around 1000 BCE, cannabis was used as a digestive, appetite stimulant, and antispasmodic to treat colic and diarrhea.[1] More recently in Europe, according to an 1890 article published in the prestigious British journal *The Lancet*, cannabis was considered "a true sedative to the stomach without causing any of the inconveniences experienced after the administration of opium, chloral, or the bromides."[2]

The endocannabinoid system (ECS), which is explained in detail in Chapter 2, plays a huge role in maintaining the health of our body's systems, including our gastrointestinal system. The ECS regulates GI motility, acid secretion, digestion, inflammation, appetite, and even nausea and vomiting. A deficiency or imbalance in our ECS can wreak havoc with our stomach and intestines. Cannabis can fill the gap, restore balance in our ECS, and help relieve some common GI problems.

GERD (GASTROESOPHAGEAL REFLUX DISEASE)

GERD (aka reflux) is the most common GI problem in the United States, affecting between 44 and more than 50 percent of adults at some point in their lives.[3] Normally the result of an overproduction of gastric acid, GERD can cause such unpleasant symptoms as heartburn, food regurgitation, nausea, hoarseness, and even tooth erosion. Diet, smoking, being overweight, and certain medications are the most common culprits.

COMMON MEDICATIONS THAT CAN CAUSE GERD

- Antibiotics
- Antihistamines
- Asthma medications
- Beta-blockers (for high blood pressure)
- Oral osteoporosis drugs, including Fosamax, Boniva, and Actonel
- Painkillers such as aspirin, ibuprofen (Advil), and naproxen (Aleve)
- Potassium supplements
- Sedatives and antidepressants

Conventional Treatment for GERD

The most frequently used treatments for GERD include OTC antacids, proton pump inhibitors (PPIs) such as omeprazole (Prilosec), and H2 blockers, including famotidine (Pepcid) and cimetidine (Tagamet). However, long-term use of H2 blockers can interfere with calcium absorption, reduce bone density, and increase the risk of hip fractures.[4] And excessive or long-term use of PPIs has also been associated with osteoporosis and bone fractures, as well as with pneumonia, cardiovascular disorders, kidney diseases, and even dementia.[5] There's also evidence that PPIs may increase the risk of *Clostridium difficile* (aka *C. diff*), a serious infection that can cause severe pain and diarrhea. *C. diff* kills about fifteen thousand people each year in the United States, most of whom are older adults.[6] Although OTC antacids may be safer, long-term use can cause diarrhea or constipation, and excessive, long-term use of antacids that contain calcium, magnesium, or aluminum can result in a buildup of these substances, which can lead to osteoporosis, kidney stones, and even kidney failure.[7]

Cannabis Treatment for GERD

Many reflux sufferers are now dumping their antacids, PPIs, and other drugs in favor of marijuana in states where it's legal. A recent study in Colorado looked at the use of these drugs before and after pot was legalized.[8] The researchers found a significant reduction in the use of conventional GERD medications after marijuana dispensaries opened in the state, an indication that patients are substituting cannabis for conventional meds. This is yet another example of the substitution effect, which has also been reported in people suffering from chronic pain, sleep problems, and mood disorders (see Chapters 4 and 5).

The medical evidence for the benefits of cannabis for GERD is becoming increasingly clear. Numerous animal studies—and some human ones as well—have demonstrated that cannabis can decrease the secretion of gastric acid while increasing the production of protective gastric mucus.[9] There's an abundance of anecdotal evidence and results from patient surveys that confirm that people suffering from GERD—as well as other GI problems—are definitely finding relief with medical marijuana.[10]

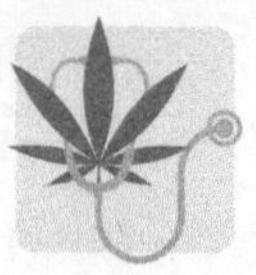

At seventy-one, Bill, an engineer, started developing persistent acid reflux and abdominal pain. He spent thousands of dollars on complementary treatments such as acupuncture and various stress management techniques. He also tried different diets (low-carb/high-fat, gluten-free, and vegetarian) and intermittent fasting. Although he wanted to avoid taking prescription medications, when his reflux worsened, he decided to try PPIs and several other drugs that his gastroenterologist recommended, none of which worked very well. When I first saw him, Bill was already on a healthy plant-based diet and was taking several GI-supportive supplements, so I decided to start him on a small dose of THC capsules three times a day with each meal. Within four weeks, all of Bill's GI symptoms completely resolved. He ultimately was able to cut down to two THC capsules twice a day. After we discussed the pros and cons of continuing, Bill decided not to risk stopping altogether.

Dr. Kogan's Cannabis Recommendations for GERD

For most GERD and other GI patients, I recommend that they follow my marijuana mantras "Start low, go slow" and "Put it where it needs to go." Oral cannabis goes directly to the GI system, unlike other routes of delivery, especially inhaling, that take a more circuitous

DIETARY AND LIFESTYLE APPROACHES TO GERD

- Avoid spicy, fatty, and acidic foods.
- Eat smaller meals slowly and chew food well.
- Don't eat two to three hours before naps or bedtime.
- Cut down on alcohol.
- Quit smoking.
- Elevate the head of your bed.
- Try some natural supplements such as rice bran oil, slippery elm, aloe vera juice, and DGL (deglycyrrhizinated licorice).

route. Coated oral capsules or chewable forms of THC taken with each meal are best for GERD and other upper GI problems. They can also help with motility issues, such as gastroparesis—a condition in which the stomach doesn't empty properly and that can actually cause GERD, as well as nausea and vomiting. Microdosing (e.g., taking a very low dose of THC, 1 mg or sometimes even less) can often be very beneficial for this and some other conditions. Plus, such a low dose is unlikely to cause any side effects and tends to cost very little.

Patients often ask me about using CBD oil for reflux, but I haven't found it very effective for either GERD or any upper GI problems. That said, if stress and anxiety are contributing to your GI problems, CBD can be helpful because of its anti-anxiety properties (see Chapter 5). And mind/body techniques can help with both the anxiety and GERD. Last but definitely not least, dietary and other lifestyle changes are essential for relieving reflux.

IBS (IRRITABLE BOWEL SYNDROME)

IBS (aka colitis or spastic colon) is a very common condition that affects up to 45 million people in the United States, most of whom are women under the age of fifty.[11] In fact, it's the most frequent problem

SIBO

SIBO (small intestinal bacterial overgrowth) is a very common cause of bloating, gas, belching, abdominal pain, diarrhea, and constipation. It's often missed, misdiagnosed, or mistreated. SIBO treatment often involves antimicrobial herbs or antibiotics, and dietary changes, especially a low FODMAP diet (a diet low in certain sugars that may cause intestinal distress).[13] Ginger and senna can also help improve GI motility. And in some cases, a low dose of THC can have a rapid and profound effect in speeding up slow motility.

diagnosed by GI doctors in the United States.[12] Rather than being a specific disease, IBS is a "functional" condition in which the bowel system fails to work well. As a result, food moves too quickly or slowly through the intestines, causing recurrent, alternate bouts of diarrhea and constipation, as well as stomach pain and bloating. Because these symptoms are also seen in several other GI conditions, especially SIBO (small intestinal bacterial overgrowth), IBS is often misdiagnosed.

Conventional Treatment for IBS

Dietary modifications, especially a high-fiber diet, can help improve symptoms. Some people also find relief from a gluten-free or low-FODMAP diet. However, most people turn to OTC and prescription medicines for their IBS symptoms, especially constipation, pain, diarrhea, and bloating. Diarrhea is arguably the most disturbing symptom because of its unpredictability and accompanying pain. OTC drugs such as Kaopectate, Pepto-Bismol, and Imodium may slow down diarrhea, but they usually don't do much to help relieve bloating and stomach pain. In fact, many OTC drugs can *cause* bloating and stomach cramps, as well as constipation, dry mouth, and dizziness.

IBS patients are often prescribed antispasmodics and antidepressants, and occasionally antibiotics. Antispasmodics are thought to help control the painful muscle spasms in the GI tract that many IBS sufferers experience. But they're not very effective and have a number of unpleasant side effects, including constipation, dry mouth, and blurry vision. Antidepressants, which are believed to have pain-relieving qualities, are often prescribed at low doses, even to patients who aren't depressed. Again, there's not much evidence that they help, and they, too, can also have disturbing side effects, including nausea, reduced appetite, insomnia, and palpitations. Antibiotics, which may be recommended for severe cases of diarrhea, can themselves cause GI problems, and their overuse can lead to antibiotic resistance and *Clostridium difficile* (*C. diff*). A relatively new antibiotic, rifaximin, has become quite popular. However, in addition to its typical side effects, it's also extremely expensive, as are some of the other new potent drugs that have recently come on the market.

Cannabis for IBS

Conventional drugs not only have unpleasant and potentially serious side effects, but the majority of patients don't find them very helpful.[14] On the other hand, IBS sufferers who turn to medical marijuana tend to be happy with the results. This is understandable. IBS—like GERD and other GI problems—is thought to be caused by an endocannabinoid deficiency or imbalance. By activating the appropriate receptors in the ECS, cannabis can help restore balance and improve gastric motility, propulsion, hypersensitivity, and inflammation.[15] In other words, pot can potentially help relieve the most common, annoying IBS symptoms. And research is beginning to confirm that it actually can.

So far, however, there have only been a few clinical studies on the effects of cannabis on IBS. One of the few studies used dronabinol,

POT IN THE PAST

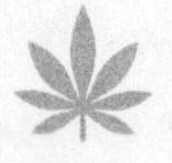

Cannabis was one of the first effective treatments for severe diarrhea caused by the cholera epidemic in the nineteenth century.[16]

the FDA-approved synthetic cannabinoid (see Chapter 2). The study found that dronabinol helped relieve diarrhea by slowing down the speed and intensity of colon contractions.[17]

There is also ample anecdotal evidence from both patients and physicians that medical marijuana helps diarrhea and other IBS symptoms.

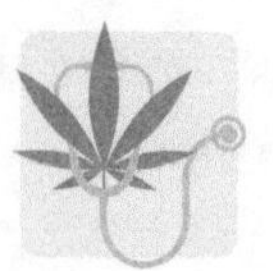

Lisa, a forty-one-year-old Washington, DC, lawyer, had been suffering from IBS for half her life, and things were getting worse. Her job required frequent trips around the country and abroad, and dealing with frequent diarrhea and severe stomach pain made these trips extremely hard. She meticulously followed a special IBS diet and tried magnesium citrate, herbal tinctures, acupuncture, craniosacral and visceral manipulation, meditation, and Epsom salt baths, all of which gave her some temporary relief. But Lisa was desperate for a permanent solution and consulted me. Since nothing else had worked, I suggested that she try cannabis, which was legal in DC. Lisa's friends had previously suggested that she try marijuana, but she had had a bad experience with it in college; she became very high and paranoid after smoking pot at a party and was hesitant to try it again. After discussing it with me, she decided to give it a go. "Start low, go slow" is one of my favorite marijuana mantras, so I started her on a very low oral dose of THC. Unfortunately, it didn't help. I then recommended that she try sublingual drops of THC and CBD, but that, too, failed. Next, I suggested that she

vape a combination of THC and CBD, which helped substantially. But Lisa disliked the side effects of vaping; they were similar to those she experienced at the college pot party—feeling uncomfortably high and paranoid. "Put it where it needs to go" is another one of my favorite marijuana mantras, so I recommended that Lisa apply a high concentration of THC/cayenne/cinnamon cream over her upper abdomen two to three times daily. Most of her symptoms were relieved after the first application! She has since been able to use a lower topical dose once a day and has remained symptom-free. During her follow-up visit, she said to me, "I wish I would have listened to some of my friends who suggested that I try marijuana years ago," and thanked me for finding the right formulation, dosage, and route and "for giving me my life back."

Dr. Kogan's Cannabis Recommendations for IBS

As mentioned above, many cases of IBS are actually misdiagnosed. But patients who have true IBS can benefit from any type or combination of cannabinoids. Though most patients prefer smoking or vaping, I encourage them to switch to the more precise oral or sublingual forms of THC, which go directly to the gut. The same mantras that applied to GERD apply to IBS as well: "Start low, go slow" and "Put it where it needs to go."

I usually start a patient on a small dose of sublingual or oral THC-predominant full-extract cannabis oil (FECO) that is high in the terpene β-caryophyllene (see Chapter 2). This can be especially helpful because it has digestive, antispasmodic, and anti-inflammatory effects, but it doesn't cause sedation or overstimulation.

Oral FECO containing 1 to 2 mg of THC two to three times a day is a safe place to start and can work well for many patients. If necessary, the dose can be slowly titrated up. For patients with predominantly

DIY FECO CAPS

Unfortunately, FECO capsules are not commonly available in dispensaries, but they are easy to make yourself. Buy empty capsules and fill them with one to two or more drops of FECO to get the appropriate dose of THC. Then fill the rest of the capsule with olive oil, or just leave it partially empty.

slow motility and constipation, I suggest starting with enteric-coated capsules of FECO containing 0.5 to 1 mg of THC with meals and, if needed, slowly increasing up to 5 mg with each meal.

Some of my patients have reported significant IBS improvement with using teas or infusions of raw cannabis. They release a very small amount of THC, while retaining all the other important ingredients in the plant, including THCa, CBDa, terpenes, and flavonoids (see Chapter 2). The healing power of the whole plant used in this way can't be underestimated. Because the gut is the target organ, teas are an excellent choice for some IBS patients. So they may be worth a try.

While oral forms of cannabis can help with IBS and some other GI problems, rectal suppositories can also be a great option (see Chapter 3). They have few side effects and are another good way to "Put it where it needs to go." Topical creams that contain a combination of THC and spices, like the one Lisa used (see above), are another possible option. They can be applied directly over the area of the abdomen that has the most symptoms. Combinations of THC or CBD, cayenne, and menthol are increasingly available in dispensaries and sold under such names as "Hot and Icy." I haven't seen consistent results with these topical creams, though, so it's not usually my first choice for most IBS patients.

Stress is a major contributing factor to IBS flare-ups and symptom intensity. Therefore, stress reduction is key to both preventing flare-ups and relieving symptoms. Diet, exercise, and other lifestyle changes

INTEGRATIVE APPROACHES TO IBS

- Probiotics
- Acupuncture
- Diet (high-fiber, gluten-free, anti-inflammatory, and low-FODMAP)
- Stress reduction (biofeedback, mindfulness, and breathing exercises, etc.)
- Exercise (moderate weight bearing and strength building, swimming, yoga, etc.)
- Peppermint, ginger, fennel, and chamomile tea
- Cognitive behavioral therapy and hypnotherapy

and integrative approaches have been proven effective in preventing and relieving the symptoms of both IBS and IBD.[18]

INFLAMMATORY BOWEL DISEASE (IBD)

IBD is much less common but more serious than IBS. Understandably, the two are often confused with each other. Although their abbreviations and symptoms are similar, they're two distinct conditions. As we mentioned above, IBS is a functional bowel disorder, while IBD is a chronic, autoimmune "structural" disease: the body's immune system mistakenly attacks and destroys healthy structures and tissues in the GI system, causing inflammation and damage to the lining of the GI tract.

IBD affects approximately 3 million people in the United States[19] and tends to strike younger people, usually under the age of thirty-five.[20] Unlike IBS, IBD affects men and women equally. It also has a genetic component; those with Northern European and Ashkenazi Jewish backgrounds are at the highest risk. There are two forms of IBD: Crohn's disease (CD), which affects the entire GI tract, and ulcerative colitis (UC), which affects only the colon. Symptoms of both may include severe diarrhea, bloody stools, stomach pain, fatigue, weight loss, and fever, which can come and go unpredictably, with varying severity. In general, Crohn's is considered the more serious of the two; 75 percent of people with CD will require surgery at some point, compared with 23 to 45 percent of people with UC.[21]

Conventional Treatment for IBD

The same OTC anti-diarrhea and antispasmodic drugs used to treat IBS are also popular with IBD patients. Although they may help somewhat, the side effects can be troublesome. To control inflammation and pain, some try ibuprofen, naproxen, and aspirin, or other NSAIDs. But even if effective, such medications can worsen IBD symptoms. As a result, most IBD patients wind up taking more potent prescription drugs.

Corticosteroids (aka steroids) such as prednisone and hydrocortisone are among the most commonly used prescription drugs. Even though they can be very effective in relieving IBD symptoms by reducing inflammation, these steroids should not be used for longer than three months.[22] Prolonged use can cause weight gain, diabetes, glaucoma, increased blood pressure, osteoporosis, and an increased risk of infections.

Mesalamine, another type of anti-inflammatory, has fewer side effects than steroids. Unfortunately, it's not very effective for Crohn's disease or the severe symptoms of ulcerative colitis.[23] Antibiotics such as Cipro and Flagyl are also frequently used to control IBD symptoms. However, as mentioned earlier in this chapter, antibiotics can worsen GI problems, and their overuse can lead to antibiotic resistance and *Clostridium difficile.*

Immunosuppressors (aka immunomodulators), such as Methotrexate, are used to treat IBD patients with severe symptoms by

WARNING!

IBD patients who take a lot of antibiotics are at increased risk of developing *Clostridium difficile* and tend to have worse outcomes than other patients who develop *C. diff.*[24] Although PPIs can increase the risk, as we mentioned above, it's the overuse or misuse of antibiotics that's now the leading cause of *C. diff* diarrhea. The use of some immunosuppressants, especially steroids, also puts IBD patients at increased risk for *C. diff.*[25]

suppressing their immune systems. This helps reduce inflammation in the intestines and lessen the need for steroids. But suppressing the immune system can cause its own serious problems, including an increased risk of infections; severe mouth sores; liver, lung, and pancreatic problems; and even some cancers.[26]

Biologics such as Humira are the newest IBD drugs on the market—and heavily promoted on TV. Biologics, which need to be injected, also help reduce inflammation. Considered more effective and safer than steroids, they come with a heavy price tag, both literally and figuratively: they have serious potential side effects, such as severe infections and some cancers, and without insurance, they can set a patient back $5,000 a month, or even more.[27] And insurance may only pay a fraction of the cost. Although biologics are being touted by both the pharmaceutical industry and physicians alike as miracle drugs for IBD, not all patients agree. According to one study, more than half of those who used them quit treatment after one year because of the side effects and/or dissatisfaction with the treatment results.[28] The high cost and the need to self-inject are other reasons patients are not big fans of biologics. Many IBD sufferers wind up seeking alternative treatments. In fact, up to 60 percent of people with IBD turn to complementary and alternative medical treatments, including herbs, acupuncture, mind/body therapies, and medical marijuana.[29]

Cannabis Treatment for IBD

Like many IBS patients, dissatisfied IBD patients are also heading to head shops to buy marijuana for relief from their often-debilitating symptoms. It's estimated that up to 40 percent of IBD patients use cannabis medically.[30]

While there have been several clinical studies on the use of pharmaceutical cannabinoids for IBS, such studies are sorely lacking for IBD. But because IBS and IBD have similar symptoms, researchers believe that if cannabinoids can help IBS patients, they can help IBD patients as well.[31] There have been a few promising small clinical studies, as well as large observational studies and surveys, on the effects of medical marijuana for IBD, most of which involved inhaled pot, and they concluded that vaping THC helped relieve patients' symptoms and improved their quality of life.[32] Most subjects also reported only minor, if any, side effects.

One small survey found that the overwhelming majority of IBD patients who used medical marijuana said that it helped relieve their symptoms, especially stomach pain.[33] A recent, large observational study of Crohn's disease patients found that those who used weed were significantly less likely than the nonusers to have serious disease complications, such as abscesses and fistulas. They also required fewer invasive procedures, including transfusions and surgery.[34]

A 2020 review article evaluated surveys and the few clinical studies that have been conducted on the use of THC for IBD. The authors concluded that "[c]annabis could have some therapeutic potential. Cannabis is particularly helpful in alleviating symptoms such as cramping, abdominal pain, and diarrhea. Patients also report an improvement of overall well-being."[35] Although some patients experienced short-term side effects, none reported significant adverse effects.

WARNING!

Most IBD patients, whether or not they use medical cannabis, go through multiple cycles of active disease and remission. If they feel normal during remission, they may feel tempted to go off their medications. But tapering off and discontinuing standard medical treatment must be done under the strict guidance of a physician. In my experience, even with a physician's guidance, only a minority of patients are able to go off their meds successfully.

Dr. Kogan's Cannabis Recommendations for IBD

While medical cannabis can help relieve IBD symptoms in some people, it's extremely important that anyone with IBD who wants to try it should first discuss it with their gastroenterologist or whoever is managing their condition. Ideally, your doctor should not only be fully informed about your intentions but be willing to work with you to include cannabis as part of your treatment protocol.

Determining what form of cannabis IBD patients should take depends on what symptoms they find most troubling. Because IBD is basically an inflammatory disease, CBD—which has anti-inflammatory properties—can be especially helpful. It also has anti-anxiety effects, which can help relieve stress and, as we've mentioned, is a very common component of IBD and other GI problems. And because most IBD patients suffer from such GI symptoms as abdominal pain, diarrhea, bloating, nausea, and vomiting, THC is equally important.

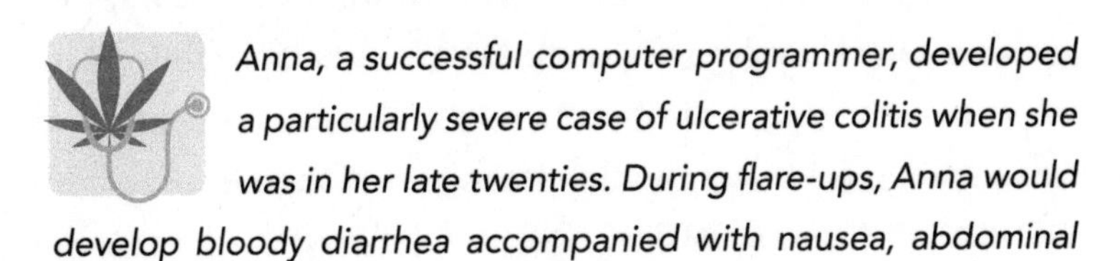

Anna, a successful computer programmer, developed a particularly severe case of ulcerative colitis when she was in her late twenties. During flare-ups, Anna would develop bloody diarrhea accompanied with nausea, abdominal

cramps, and severe fatigue. By the time she was in her early thirties, Anna was told that she would likely need surgery to remove her entire colon. Between flare-ups, she often felt reasonably well. But Anna still had several severe flares each year that required changes in her steroids and other medications. The prospect of losing her colon pushed Anna to seek alternative approaches.

When Anna first saw me, we decided to proceed with a trial of high-dose oral and rectal probiotics, acupuncture, and a number of anti-inflammatory dietary changes and supplements. While this definitely helped with the severity of the flares, they still occurred regularly. We next decided to try controlling the nausea and abdominal pain during her flare-ups with sublingual cannabis oil and vaping flower high in THC. While this helped somewhat, it didn't decrease the severity or frequency of the flares. So I decided to start her on rectal suppositories and chose a ratio of 1:1 THC:CBD, starting with 5 mg total of THC and CBD. This dose optimized the anti-inflammatory effects of CBD, while still assuring a high enough dose of THC to relieve her pain. After reaching a total dose of 25 mg each of THC and CBD twice daily, her flares had stopped altogether. During the past several years, Anna had only one mild flare-up, which was controlled with a short course of prednisone.

While Anna's case may appear to be rather remarkable, it's not unique. I've had several other patients who have used rectal suppositories for both Crohn's disease and ulcerative colitis and have achieved dramatic benefits.

The route of delivery is definitely key and will depend mostly on where the disease is located. For example, if someone has ulcerative colitis with rectal involvement, rectal cannabis suppositories would be by far the first choice. If the patient also has abdominal pain and nausea, I would start them with a low-potency suppository of 5 mg 1:1:1 THC:CBD:CBDa or 1:1 THC:CBD combined with a low 1 to 2 mg sublingual dose of THC twice daily. CBDa is a potent anti-inflammatory and analgesic (see Chapter 2). If the pain and nausea become severe, occasionally inhaling THC-predominant flower can be helpful. However, if someone has Crohn's disease that affects the upper intestinal tract, the oral route is best. I suggest that they take cannabis capsules starting at 1 mg, titrating slowly up to as much as is needed, which often can be a rather high dose of 10 mg several times a day. Similar to my recommendations for rectal suppositories, I suggest a ratio of 1:1:1 THC:CBD:CBDa.

As we have mentioned throughout this chapter, dietary and other lifestyle approaches—especially stress reduction—are extremely important when dealing with GI problems. While the addition of medical marijuana may not work miracles, it can go a long way in helping relieve reflux, IBS, and IBD. And it can help you to de-stress as well!

MARIJUANA AND MORNING SICKNESS

Increasing numbers of pregnant women are using pot during pregnancy; estimates run as high as 35 percent during the first trimester, outpacing the use of cannabis by nonpregnant women,[36] and it's believed that morning sickness is the motivating factor. Between 70 and 80 percent of pregnant women experience morning sickness or other prolonged bouts of nausea and vomiting.[37] And most report that these symptoms have a profoundly negative effect on their physical, emotional, and professional lives. Because there's substantial evidence that cannabis is safe and effective in treating chemo-related nausea and vomiting, it's assumed that cannabis can also help relieve pregnancy-related nausea and vomiting. Small studies and surveys bear this out,[38] but that doesn't mean it's safe to use cannabis while pregnant (or breastfeeding).

Some epidemiological studies associate cannabis use during pregnancy with premature births, low-birth-weight babies, and miscarriages.[39] (We should note that in at least one of the studies, other behaviors such as smoking and drinking during pregnancy appeared to be contributing factors.[40]) However, there's much clearer evidence that prescription nausea- and vomiting-reducing drugs (antiemetics) cause severe birth defects. Think of thalidomide, the drug used in the 1950s and early '60s to treat pregnancy-related nausea and vomiting that was responsible for thousands of babies being born with severe birth defects. Since then, other antiemetics used by pregnant women have also caused birth defects.[41]

So even though cannabis can be effective for nausea and vomiting, we don't recommend it to pregnant women because of the possible risks to the fetus. That said, we recognize that in some cases of severe nausea and vomiting, when other alternatives don't work, a sublingual form of cannabis might be indicated (this would circumvent the dangers of inhaling). On the other hand, cannabis edibles are not a great idea for someone suffering from nausea and vomiting.

Several years ago, I was called in to consult on a pregnant patient who was admitted to the hospital for such severe vomiting that her doctors feared that it could trigger premature labor, putting her fetus's life at risk. They tried all kinds of medications to no avail and the patient said she wanted to try marijuana. The initial response from the staff was very negative, but I helped them come around. We started her on inhaled cannabis, which was very effective. After a week, her vomiting was controlled, her nausea improved, and we were able to switch her to sublingual drops. I also insisted she add CBD to minimize any possible risk to the baby's developing brain that THC might cause.

Although randomized clinical studies could help determine if cannabis use is safe during pregnancy, such studies would be unethical because of the potential risks to the fetus and offspring. However, there are longitudinal studies of women who use pot during pregnancy in the works that could help clarify the matter.[42] In the meantime, it's better to be safe than sorry.

CHAPTER SEVEN

Skin Problems

Skin—which includes hair and nails—is our largest organ, covering every visible part of our body except our eyeballs and teeth. Because skin problems are difficult to hide, they can cause undue damage to our self-esteem. It's no wonder skin-care products are a multibillion-dollar industry. And cannabis-infused products are a growing part of that industry, with loads of moisturizers, wrinkle reducers, sunscreens, lubricants, and dandruff treatments for sale.

But skin problems are more than cosmetic concerns; they can cause intense itching, physical pain, and emotional suffering. Moreover, they can be the result of a number of medical and other factors that require more attention than simply addressing what you see in the mirror. For example, acne, eczema, psoriasis, and herpes are mostly the result of systemic or internal problems, while skin allergies, fungal infections, and skin cancer are often caused by external, environmental assaults. And genetics, emotions, and lifestyle play key roles as well.

The endocannabinoid system (ECS) also plays an important role in maintaining the health of our skin as well as of all our body's other systems and organs (see Chapter 2). When our ECS gets out of whack from hormonal changes, diet, and environmental toxins, among other causes, our skin can pay the price. The unfortunate results: everything from atopic dermatitis to zits. By stimulating appropriate receptors in the ECS, topical cannabinoids can help restore our skin's health. Increasing scientific evidence confirms that cannabis can help treat a number of skin disorders, including acne, eczema, psoriasis, herpes, and even skin cancer.[1] And topical cannabis is the most direct, most effective, and easiest way to do so (see Chapter 2). It's also a great example of my marijuana mantra "Put it where it needs to go."

ACNE

Acne is the most common skin disorder in the world, affecting more than 50 million people in the United States alone. Acne is an inflammatory process that involves chronic skin infections primarily caused by bacteria. Hormones are the major culprits; pimples are most likely to pop up as we age, especially during puberty, periods, pregnancy, and peri- and postmenopause. Diet, stress, skin products, and even genes can cause or exacerbate this unattractive, unwelcome problem. Acne occurs when the sebaceous glands—which secrete an oily substance (sebum)—get inflamed and become clogged with dirt, bacteria, dead skin, or oil, causing pimples to pop out. These glands also get overstimulated by hormonal changes and so produce more sebum . . . and pimples.

Conventional Treatment for Acne

There's a wide array of OTC and prescription drugs for acne that work with varying degrees of success. Rx steroids are among the more successful treatments. But long-term use can cause topical steroid addiction and withdrawal syndrome (aka red skin syndrome), a condition in which patients who discontinue treatment start to experience disturbing symptoms, including stinging, burning, and extreme redness.[2]

And some antibiotics, hormones, and other Rx drugs have been linked to such serious conditions as liver damage, blood clots, severe depression, and birth defects in offspring. Unfortunately, people with severe acne throw out thousands of dollars on these potentially dangerous drugs as well as on often useless OTC products. Medical marijuana offers acne sufferers a safer and possibly more effective way to zap zits.

Cannabis Treatment for Acne

Cannabis interacts with ECS receptors to help restore skin health; it has anti-inflammatory effects on the sebaceous glands, inhibits oil production, and prevents the spread of acne.[3] Because of these effects—which have recently been dubbed the "anti-acne trinity"—cannabis is now recognized as a very promising, safe, effective, and cost-effective treatment for severe acne.[4]

Although there have been very few clinical studies, a recent small one found that 3 percent cannabis seed extract cream was helpful in reducing acne-related skin oiliness and redness.[5] Both inhaled and topical forms of cannabis have been shown to be effective, but topical is preferable.

According to the American Academy of Dermatology (AAD), there are no negative effects from the topical use of cannabis except for occasional contact dermatitis, which could be a side effect from any topical substance. In fact, the AAD explains that contact dermatitis from topical cannabis is more likely to be caused by some added ingredient rather than the cannabis itself.[6] To be safe, it's best to apply the cannabis to a small section of your skin before applying it to a large area.

WARNING!

Although acne most commonly affects teenagers and young adults, these groups should avoid using medical marijuana. THC has been shown to have a detrimental effect on growing brains, although it's not clear that topical THC would affect them as much as smoked, vaped, or edible forms. Still, it's better to be safe than sorry and to wait until the early twenties before using medical marijuana for acne or other conditions. If nothing else has worked, and cannabis is the only remaining option, anyone under twenty-one should use topical cream that is predominantly CBD, ideally 10:1 CBD:THC.

Dr. Kogan's Cannabis Recommendations for Acne

Although data is limited, applying THC creams, lotions, or soaps on the face can very possibly produce unwanted psychoactive effects. To reduce this risk, I suggest you start with a topical application of 1:1 THC:CBD. Another option is to start with a high concentration of cannabis- or hemp-derived CBD cream or salve. A number of my patients claim that hemp-based topicals helped their acne. As mentioned above, bacteria are a major cause of acne. Both CBD and THC are known to have some antibacterial properties, which may explain—at least in part—their anti-acne effect.[7] There are several pharmaceutical companies developing CBD-based topical acne creams, so the future may determine what is the most efficacious. In fact, there have been some recent clinical trials using a synthetic topical CBD (BTX 1503) for severe acne.[8] So far, the drug has been effective in reducing the number of lesions. However, if and when approved by the FDA, the cost is bound to be sky-high. At this point in time, most dispensaries already sell natural THC and CBD topicals at a reasonable price.

In any case, stick with a non-scented, hypoallergenic cannabis product made from natural ingredients and natural preservatives—

DIY TOPICALS

Unfortunately, cannabis-infused shampoos, soaps, and lotions are harder to find and tend to be pricier than cannabis creams and gels. The good news is you can make your own at home by mixing THC with aloe vera gel, shea or cocoa butter, and vitamin E oil. There are also some online resources for making your own topical products listed in Appendix II: Cannabis Resources.

such as vitamin E—and avoid other chemical additives. For any topical concerns, it's a good idea to perform a patch test before using by applying a small amount on the affected area twice a day for a few days before extending to a larger area. For severe cases, THC:CBD shampoos, soaps, or lotions can also be helpful, along with—or in place of—topical applications.

The most recent addition to my skin recommendations for acne (and psoriasis) is topical CBG. Similar to CBD, CBG is a potent anti-inflammatory (see Chapter 2). Although my experience is limited, I've already seen good results, especially when topical CBG is combined with topical CBD and THC.

ORAL HERPES (HSV-1)

Whether it's called cold sores or fever blisters, most of us have suffered from this unsightly, painful condition. Medically known as herpes simplex virus 1 or HSV-1, this form of herpes mostly affects the mouth but can erupt anywhere on the face and body. This is different from herpes simplex 2 or HSV-2, which typically affects the genitals. Most people in the United States are infected with the herpes HSV-1 virus by the age of twenty. After the first infection, the virus becomes dormant in the nerve tissues. Certain triggers—such as fevers, stress, and physical injury—can reactivate the virus and cause cold sores. All forms of herpes are highly contagious and there is no cure. Once the virus is in your body, it's there to stay. While most herpes flare-ups can be painful as well as cosmetically disturbing, the blisters usually go away in a week or so. But, unfortunately, herpes not only can leave scars, it's likely to reoccur . . . often at the most inopportune times.

Conventional Treatment for Herpes

There are countless OTC treatments for herpes that can help dry up the blisters and kill the pain. Although, so far, nothing has been able to totally kill the virus, there are a number of antiviral prescription tablets and topicals that help hasten the healing and prevent the herpes from spreading. But the oral drugs all have potential side effects, including dizziness, headache, gastrointestinal problems, and joint pain, to name a few.

Cannabis Treatment for Herpes

Since 1980, several laboratory studies have demonstrated that THC has antiviral effects and may be helpful in the treatment of herpes simplex.[9] But clinical studies are sorely lacking because of the Schedule I status of cannabis, which makes it federally illegal (see Chapter 2). In addition, oral herpes is not considered a very serious problem—at least to the scientific community. Unlike acne, eczema, and psoriasis, the blisters are small and localized and usually disappear in a week or so.

Although we might have to wait awhile for evidence from clinical studies, the anecdotal evidence from patients and physicians is very convincing. In fact, I can personally vouch for the benefits of THC for treating and preventing oral herpes.

For decades I've suffered from painful cold sores on my lower lip, which would worsen during the winter. My cold sores would continuously crack and bleed in cold weather and never fully heal, even in warm months. Although the actual flare-ups of herpes were not that frequent, my cracked lip would not heal completely between episodes, especially in the winter. While a relatively minor problem that was mostly a cosmetic issue, every dentist I went to mentioned it. Finally, I paid attention when one dentist warned me that recurrent oral herpes could lead to lip cancer. It concerned me enough to try every conventional and alternative treatment I could find, including antiviral creams, different types of OTC lip ointments, and tea tree oil and other herbal remedies. Unfortunately, nothing worked. During one of my flare-ups, a colleague gave me a standard size lip balm of 100 mg of pure THC. I used it three times a day, and in two weeks the herpes was completely gone! That was years ago, and I have not had any recurrences. However, to be on the safe side, I still use the THC lip balm during the winter months. One lip balm lasts me for many months since very little needs to be applied at a time.

Dr. Kogan's Cannabis Recommendations for Herpes

For HSV-1 outbreaks, I recommend applying pure topical THC as often as every two to three hours during the first few days and to keep applying it two to three times a day for at least four weeks after the skin completely heals. If you can find them, THC lip balms are definitely the best option for cold sores on your lips. If you can't find them, you can make your own by mixing 100 mg of THC with beeswax, shea butter, or coconut oil.

If you live in a state that hasn't yet legalized medical marijuana, try hemp-derived CBD cream, which is widely available in stores or online. If an outbreak is very severe and lesions are not healing quickly, seek medical attention. Applying topical cannabis or anything else directly to larger open wounds is *not* advisable. Open wounds require specialized treatments.

WARNING!

If you or a friend has oral herpes, don't share joints, vaping devices, edibles, or THC lip balms. Oral herpes is highly transmissible!

As with acne and psoriasis, especially if THC is not available, try topical CBG or a CBD:CBG mixture. Again, always look for full-extract products rather than isolates to get the benefits of the entourage effect (see Chapter 2).

ECZEMA (ATOPIC DERMATITIS)

Eczema (aka atopic dermatitis), which is often thought of as a childhood disease, affects approximately 16.5 million adults in the United States.[10] Itchy, dry, scaly, cracked, and painful red skin are the hallmarks of eczema. The most common areas affected are the face, hands, feet, behind the knees, and in the elbow joints.

Eczema is a chronic inflammatory condition that comes and goes. The flare-ups are often caused by stress, anxiety, and diet. People with eczema frequently suffer from self-consciousness and embarrassment, especially when it affects the face. In addition to the cosmetic concerns, many eczema sufferers are especially bothered by pain and severe itchiness. But the majority are never diagnosed by physicians[11] and tend to seek relief from OTC steroids and other topical products, which are often ineffective.

The exact cause of eczema, which often runs in families, is unknown. It's believed to be the result of an overactive immune system, but there's some debate as to whether it's an actual autoimmune disease. There's also evidence that the skin microbiome—the bacteria that normally live on the skin—may play an important role. The skin

MRSA AND MARIJUANA

Studies have found that cannabis, which has both antimicrobial and antibacterial properties, can be effective in killing some strains of MRSA.[12] In theory, according to a recent study, topical THC and CBD may be able to cure MSRA because they have anti-MRSA properties.[13] Given the urgent need for a cure, researchers will hopefully clarify the clinical applicability of cannabis in combating this dreadful disease in the next few years.[14]

of people with eczema is often found to have an excess of *Staphylococcus aureus* bacteria, which can be both a cause and complication of eczema. Topical forms of cannabis have been found to be helpful in both preventing and controlling this bacterium.[15] *Staphylococcus aureus* is actually the same bacterium as MRSA (methicillin-resistant *Staphylococcus aureus*), the notorious and potentially deadly bacteria that has proven so resistant to most antibiotics.

Conventional Treatment for Eczema

Although there's no cure for eczema, there are a plethora of OTC and prescription drugs and lifestyle approaches that have helped treat eczema and/or prevent flare-ups to varying degrees. Drug treatments—which typically include topical, oral, and injectable steroids and antibiotics—can sometimes be effective but long-term use has the potentially serious side effects described above, including weight gain, diabetes, glaucoma, increased blood pressure, osteoporosis, and an increased risk of infections. Overuse of topical steroids can also cause red skin syndrome (see Conventional Treatment for Acne, above). And long-term or overuse of antibiotics can lead to antibiotic resistance and even *Clostridium difficile,* a serious infection that can cause severe pain and diarrhea. The more potent biologics and immune sup-

WARNING!

Steroid creams are the most common treatment for eczema. However, the frequent and continuous use of steroids for severe eczema (or acne) can lead to an uncommon but very concerning condition called red skin syndrome (RSS) or topical steroid withdrawal syndrome (TWS). This is a condition in which steroids not only stop working but make the condition worse. The skin becomes very red and inflamed, causing intense burning and itching. For more information on RSS, check out this link: https://www.itsan.org/.

pressants, like Dupixent and methotrexate, can have even more severe adverse reactions. Because they suppress the immune system, they put patients at increased risk for infections, liver and kidney damage, and even some cancers.[16] And they can also be extremely expensive, and often require periodic monitoring for side effects. This just adds to the already high costs, which are not always covered by insurance. On top of that, they often don't work very well. Because of their lack of effectiveness and adverse effects—as well as costs and inconvenience—more than two out of three eczema patients stop using them within a year, according to a large recent study.[17]

Cannabis Treatment for Eczema

Cannabis can work extremely well for treating eczema, especially when combined with lifestyle approaches, light therapy, dietary adjustments, stress reduction, moisturizers, and warm baths. Compared with conventional medical treatments for eczema, medical marijuana and lifestyle strategies are much safer, often more effective, and usually cheaper. And they can also be more enjoyable.

Cannabis is effective in treating eczema symptoms because of

POT IN THE PAST

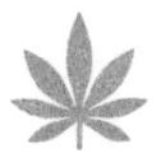

"[A] pill of cannabis indica at bedtime has at my hands sometimes afforded relief to the intolerable itching of eczema."

—Henry Granger Piffard, MD (a founder of American dermatology), 1881[18]

its anti-inflammatory, antimicrobial, and anti-pruritus (itching) properties and has been proven to be remarkably effective in relieving itching.[19] Severe itchiness is one of eczema's most disturbing and relentless symptoms. When you itch, you scratch. And scratching causes the skin to become swollen, painful, and inflamed . . . and itch even more. This vicious cycle of itching and scratching just exacerbates the problem. Both the pain and itchiness can be so severe that they interfere with sleep, daytime functioning, and quality of life. In addition to topical cannabis, a recent study found that dietary hempseed oil was helpful in reducing skin dryness and itchiness.[20]

Because eczema can be aesthetically, physiologically, and psychologically disturbing, it's not surprising that a recent survey conducted by the National Eczema Association found that almost one-third of people with eczema were diagnosed with depression and/or anxiety.[21] Stress is also common and both anxiety and stress can trigger an eczema attack—yet another vicious cycle.[22] Medical cannabis has been shown to help relieve stress, anxiety, and depression, as well as help with sleep problems (see Chapter 5).

Dr. Kogan's Cannabis Recommendations for Eczema

Although eczema can be very difficult to treat, I've had good results treating my patients with medical cannabis. I usually recommend starting out with topical full-spectrum 1:1 THC:CBD or triple topical THC:CBD:CBDa. CBDa (cannabidiolic acid) is a potent anti-inflammatory and analgesic (see Chapter 2).

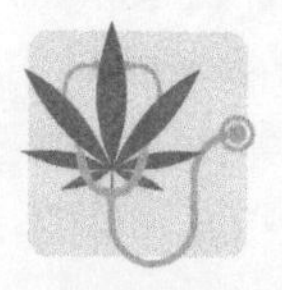

When Cindy, a thirty-seven-year-old grant writer, came to see me, she had undiagnosed severe hand and foot eczema. This was not only a cosmetic problem, it also interfered with her work; when the outbreaks were severe, her hands hurt so much that she couldn't type. She tried a variety of steroid creams and other over-the-counter remedies, but nothing worked. I recommended that she topically apply a 1:1 THC/CBD lotion and started her on an anti-inflammatory diet. I also suggested ways for her to manage her stress better, since eczema and stress are very strongly linked. At her follow-up visit twelve weeks later, her eczema symptoms were 80 percent improved! At her next follow-up, six months later, she felt and looked even better and said to me, "As long as I cope with my stressors and stay on the diet you put me on, my rash is gone! When it does come back, it reminds me that I have to readjust my lifestyle by minding my diet, reducing my stress, and using the topical THC/CBD cream you recommended, all of which completely keep the problem at bay."

My recommendations for treatment are based on how inflamed the eczema looks as well as the other symptoms. In Cindy's case, her eczema was usually dry and not very red or swollen. But because it was very itchy and at times painful, it was important that she use a topical with a high ratio of THC to CBD.

On the other hand, Karl, an eighty-one-year-old, long-term patient of mine found an excellent response from a full-spectrum hemp-based CBD salve, which completely resolved his chronic leg eczema. The cream Karl used also contained calendula, an herb that helps with a variety of chronic skin problems. Karl continues to apply a thin layer of the cream every day prophylactically, which has prevented his eczema from recurring.

Another cannabinoid, CBG (cannabigerol), is the "new kid on the block" that has become quite popular, and for good reason. CBG is a nonintoxicating cannabinoid that has been shown to reduce pain and inflammation (see Chapter 2). I've seen some excellent results when patients apply a high concentration of topical CBD:CBG cream directly on their eczema lesions two to three times a day. Unfortunately, CBG is not usually available in cannabis dispensaries, but because it's derived from hemp, CBD:CBG cream can be bought legally online. CBD:THC cream or salve can also be effective. In fact, many of my patients claim that *any* topical cannabis creams work well, including CBD alone, as long as the cannabinoid concentration is high enough. Usually, 150 mg of total cannabinoids (THC and/or CBD) per ounce of topical preparation does the trick. In general, I find that if topical cannabis is going to work for eczema, it does so rather quickly—within a few weeks.

What is rather important for eczema—and all skin conditions discussed in this chapter—is that the amount of topical cannabinoids necessary to achieve positive results is usually quite small and, therefore, cost-effective. Starting with a twice-daily application of a thin layer on the affected areas should be sufficient for most people, although for severe cases more frequent daily applications may be needed.

It's also essential that patients suffering from eczema address the issue of possible food allergies, a common trigger for outbreaks. Because gluten, dairy products, eggs, and nuts are common culprits, it's a good idea to eliminate them one at a time and see if that has any effect on the eczema. An anti-inflammatory diet may also help. (See health.harvard.edu/staying-healthy/the-best-anti-inflammatory-diets) Some patients also opt to have food-allergy testing, which can be helpful in guiding dietary modifications. And because stress often plays a huge role in flare-ups, mind/body techniques—such as meditation, yoga, biofeedback, tai chi—can help enormously. This is also good advice for patients suffering from psoriasis.

PSORIASIS

Psoriasis and eczema have a lot in common and often get confused with each other. They both involve inflammation of the skin, unsightly rashes or patches, itchiness, and sometimes pain. While they both often appear on the same parts of the body, including the face, hands, and feet, psoriasis also commonly appears on the scalp, palms, and soles of the feet. Although psoriasis affects fewer adults than eczema (6.7 million versus 16.5 million), it's a more serious and difficult condition to treat. As many as 30 percent of people with psoriasis also have or will develop psoriatic arthritis, a painful condition that causes joints to become stiff and inflamed.[23]

Psoriasis is a chronic autoimmune disease, a condition in which the body's immune system attacks its own healthy tissue or organs, mistaking them for something foreign and potentially dangerous. In psoriasis, the immune system causes the skin to grow too quickly, possibly as a way to protect itself from outside invaders. The excess skin cells build up and form thick red skin patches that are covered with silvery white patches of dead skin, which can crack and bleed (aka plaque psoriasis).

Conventional Treatment for Psoriasis

Many of the medical treatments for psoriasis are the same or similar to the treatments for eczema, including cortisone, biologics, and immunosuppressants, with the same potentially serious side effects and high costs. Some topical retinoids (vitamins A and D), salicylic acid creams, and coal tar may be helpful, but can also have some serious side effects. Light therapy, moisturizers, dandruff shampoos, and lifestyle adjustments—which are also recommended—are not only safer bets but also work well along with cannabis treatment.

Cannabis Treatment for Psoriasis

There is considerable evidence that cannabis can be an effective treatment for psoriasis.[24] It helps relieve psoriasis symptoms in the same ways it helps relieve the symptoms of eczema, especially by reducing inflammation, itching, and even stress.[25] In addition, there's evidence that cannabis slows the growth of skin cells and helps prevent their buildup on the skin.[26]

One of the most painful symptoms of psoriasis is cracked, bleeding skin, and a recent study (in mice) demonstrated that cannabis can help heal skin wounds.[27]

Dr. Kogan's Cannabis Recommendations for Psoriasis

In general, I find psoriasis a lot more difficult to control than eczema. But topical cannabis can be remarkably effective for some patients. I usually recommend that they start with pure THC cream, which usually works well. I also suggest that psoriasis patients add some CBD, because of its anti-inflammatory effects. In fact, many patients find that in addition to CBD, they get benefits from creams containing CBG or CBDa. As mentioned above, both CBG and CBDa have strong anti-inflammatory properties. But I've also seen dramatic effects from pure THC topical products.

Just after his thirtieth birthday, George, a computer programmer, started to develop small, dry patches on his face that progressively got worse. His sister currently had psoriasis, and his father told him that the same thing had happened to him when he was his age. George started using OTC steroid cream, which initially helped, but his face increasingly looked worse. He was very concerned because he and his fiancée, Debby, were planning to get married in a few months. His sister gave him her prescription steroid cream to use before his summer wedding. It kept his skin under control for the ceremony and honeymoon. But the honeymoon was soon over, and the psoriasis returned with a vengeance. As Debby graphically explained: "It looked like a really bad windburn—his skin was red and leathery, and people started commenting on how bad it looked. That caused him a lot of stress. He was also really itchy and in pain. His skin was constantly flaking, and it was now all over his body and head, not just on his face."

George went to his regular doctor, who was shocked at how bad George's skin looked. He referred George to a dermatologist, who immediately prescribed a strong cortisone cream. It helped reduce the redness but not his other, more disturbing symptoms. The dermatologist then prescribed the widely advertised immunosuppressant Otezla, which George rejected. Not only was he concerned about the side effects, which included severe depression, diarrhea, nausea, and vomiting, it was extremely expensive—up to $40,000 a year! George heard that medical marijuana could help and consulted a colleague of mine, who gave him samples of three cannabis products: THC hair oil, THC cream, and THC soap. George used the cream and oil for his skin patches, the oil for his hairy areas, and the soap for showering. Within two days, George noticed some improvement in his skin as well as on his scalp and on the areas with body hair. Over the next month, he had fewer plaques and reduced redness on his torso, face, and head. "He's so happy with how well it's working," said Debby. "We have a wedding to go to this summer, and last night he was saying how excited he is that his face is going to look normal for it." George attributed the improvement to the THC soap, which he thinks is "controlling everything." After two months of treatment, Debby reported that "George uses the hair oil only once every two weeks or so, at the first sign of his scalp getting itchy, and one use usually does the trick!" She added, "He swears by the body wash, though!"

This case was so remarkable that my colleague and I published the results in the *Journal of Drugs in Dermatology* in August 2020.[28]

TOPICAL TIPS

Topical applications of THC and other cannabinoids are often the best solutions for many skin problems, especially the ones in this chapter. In addition to following my marijuana mantra "Put it where it needs to go," it's important to follow my other favorite mantra, "Start low, go slow." Remember to apply topical cannabis on a small area of the skin first to minimize the risk of a severe allergic reaction. Also, read labels carefully and avoid artificial ingredients that are known to be harmful such as parabens, colorings, and dyes. The best topical bases are food-grade ingredients such as olive oil, shea butter, beeswax, and jojoba oil.

It's best to choose full-spectrum hemp or cannabis oils. In addition to THC and CBD, they contain a variety of other, potentially beneficial active ingredients such as terpenes, flavonoids, and fatty acids. As described in Chapter 2, terpenes are especially important; they not only give cannabis and other plants their flavor and aroma, they also enhance their medical benefits (aka the entourage effect).

CANNABIS COSMETICS

The topical tips above apply equally to cannabis cosmetics. CBD and hemp-infused skin products—including moisturizers, wrinkle reducers, hair enhancers, eye masks, and sunscreens, among others—have flooded the cosmetic market. In fact, in 2018, the global CBD skin-care market was $630 million,[29] with North America having the largest share. CBD and hemp skin-care products are sold online and in drugstores, but upscale department stores are now jumping

BUYER BEWARE!

If you're planning to buy CBD or hemp-based skin-care products, read the label carefully to avoid being fooled by a low price that seems too good to be true. Don't only look for the percentage of CBD (which may not even be listed), but also look for its location on the label. The higher up CBD is listed, the higher the concentration and potency. If CBD is near the bottom of the list, don't waste your money! And before you go to the checkout counter, check out the rest of the ingredients to rule out toxins or other undesirable or unnecessary ingredients. To help evaluate the quality of cannabis cosmetic products, go to https://www.ewg.org or https://www.consumerlab.com.

on the bandwagon. Because of the lack of regulations, consumers are spending big bucks on these products without any proof that they work or that they actually contain what they claim to. In fact, a recent study of a variety of online CBD products found that only 31 percent of the products were accurately labeled.[30]

Dermatological cannabis research is understandably focused on their benefits for skin diseases, so while the efficacy of cannabis cosmetics may someday be clarified by future research, it's not a top priority. However, research on dermatological cannabis can apply to cannabis cosmetics. For example, recent small studies—both in animals and humans—have demonstrated that topical cannabis may be effective as sunscreen lotions. Some formulations have been shown to have high levels of SPF and therefore can block dangerous UV sunrays.[31] This is especially important since skin cancer is the most common cancer in the United States and kills more than two people every hour.[32] Even more significant is compelling new evidence that cannabis may be effective for the treatment of the deadliest form of skin cancer, melanoma.[33] The role of cannabis in cancer treatment is discussed in the next chapter.

CHAPTER EIGHT

Cancer

Cancer is arguably the most dreaded diagnosis we'll ever receive. It not only terrifies us because it's a potentially painful disease with a dire prognosis, but cancer treatment—even when successful—can be dreadful. The side effects of chemotherapy and radiation—nausea, vomiting, loss of appetite, and pain—are well known. Surgery can be painful, in both the short and the long term. Most cancer patients also suffer from anxiety, depression, and insomnia because of the diagnosis, treatment, or both.[1] The benefits of medical marijuana for these side effects are also well known in the cancer community; it's estimated that between a quarter to almost half of cancer patients use medical marijuana for their cancer-related symptoms. In fact, medical cannabis is more popular among cancer patients than among the general population, and the majority of cancer patients who use medical marijuana are women over the age of fifty.[2]

Cancer, in fact, is one of the few qualifying conditions for the use of medical cannabis in states where it's legal. Still, as with the other conditions discussed in this book, clinical research is lagging behind. This is because of not only the federal laws that have hindered cannabis clinical research but the fact that much of the research on cannabis and cancer has focused on how smoking pot may *cause* lung and other cancers, rather than the role of cannabis in helping relieve cancer-related symptoms and the side effects of cancer treatment.

Medical marijuana can, in fact, be helpful for both the symptoms caused by cancer treatment and the cancer itself, sometimes simultaneously. As my colleague Dr. Donald Abrams, a world-renowned cannabis expert and oncologist, put it:

> *I frequently see people dealing with nausea, loss of appetite, pain, insomnia, and anxiety/depression. I could write prescriptions for four or five different medications, all of which might interact with each other or the cancer treatments I am using. Or I could recommend they try one intervention that can potentially take care of all of those symptoms—cannabis!*[3]

NAUSEA AND VOMITING

Nausea and vomiting are the most disruptive, disturbing, feared, and commonly reported side effects of cancer treatment. Unfortunately, up to 80 percent of patients undergoing chemotherapy experience what's medically referred to as CINV (chemotherapy-induced nausea and vomiting).[4] These distressing symptoms, which also occur in patients undergoing radiation treatment, can strike a patient during treatment or a week or longer afterward (aka delayed phase). In fact, nausea and vomiting are actually more common, more severe, and more difficult to treat in the delayed phase.[5] CINV sometimes strikes even *before* a chemo session, a phenomenon known as "anticipatory nausea and vomiting"—a conditioned response to just the mere thought of receiving chemotherapy. These and other treatment side effects can be so physically, emotionally, and socially devastating that many patients have stopped their cancer treatment—or even refused to start treatment in the first place.[6]

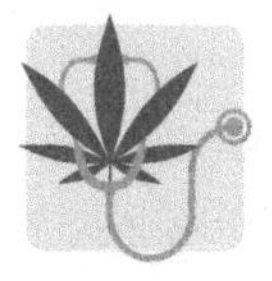

Sophia, a jewelry designer, was sixty-seven when she was diagnosed with stage IV breast cancer. She was devastated, not just about the dire diagnosis, but the prospect of having chemotherapy. "I didn't want chemo because it's the worst treatment. The side effects are disastrous. I was afraid of being really sick—throwing up for months and months. I was so concerned about getting so sick it would kill me that I decided not to have chemo."

Conventional Treatment for Nausea and Vomiting

A number of prescription anti-nausea and anti-vomiting medications (referred to as antiemetics) are frequently used before, during, or after treatment. The most common ones are corticosteroids, serotonin receptor antagonists, and neurokinin receptor antagonists.[7] Depending on the drug, side effects can range from constipation, dry mouth, insomnia, dizziness, and headaches to cardiovascular problems and allergic reactions. Paradoxically, while these antiemetics can be very helpful in preventing vomiting, they're not very effective in preventing or treating nausea. Indeed, up to 70 percent of patients suffer from nausea despite taking these drugs.[8] Unfortunately, most oncologists overestimate the effectiveness of antiemetics, which can lead to the undertreatment of their patients.[9]

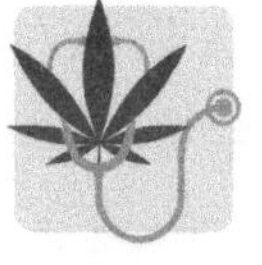

Sophia's husband persuaded her to try chemo after her doctor said that if he put her on the strongest chemo regimen, she'd have a 30 percent chance of survival, which was very high for her diagnosis. "I finally agreed. I

figured if I was gonna take a chance and take chemo, I'd take the strongest chemo. If it's gonna kill me, it's gonna kill me. It was my only option." Sophia was given antiemetics and painkillers during her treatments, but they didn't work. In fact, she said, "Anything they gave me for nausea and pain made me really, really sick. The drugs they gave me for nausea were the worst. I threw them all out! I told my doctor I didn't want any more drugs—I was gonna take medical marijuana."

Cannabis for Nausea and Vomiting

Because the endocannabinoid system (ECS) plays a role in regulating nausea and vomiting (see Chapter 2), cannabis can play an important role in preventing and treating them.[10] Physicians' reliance on conventional antiemetics is unfortunate. Cannabis (both synthetic pharmacological and natural) has been proven more effective, but it's not always offered or even available to patients.

Since 1985, two FDA-approved synthetic forms of THC, dronabinol (Marinol) and nabilone (Cesamet), have been used somewhat successfully to treat CINV. According to the highly regarded recent report by the National Academies of Sciences, Engineering, and Medicine, "There is conclusive evidence that oral cannabinoids are effective antiemetics in the treatment of chemotherapy-induced nausea and vomiting."[11] A number of studies have found that nabilone and dronabinol are even more effective than some conventional antiemetics,[12] but their adverse effects are a problem for many patients. Unfortunately, many doctors don't consider cannabinoids, much less medical marijuana, valid options for patients suffering from CINV. These doctors may be uncomfortable with the idea of their patients using any form of cannabis. And some don't offer it because of its potential psychoactive side effects, which include euphoria, drowsiness, dizziness, and disorientation.

Still, studies have consistently found that the majority of patients (up to 90 percent in some studies) prefer cannabis to other antiemetics.[13] This preference persists despite the fact that the common side effects of both synthetic and natural cannabis have been reported to be *more* intense and frequent than those of conventional antiemetics.

So why would patients prefer a drug with more side effects? It's believed that patients actually consider these so-called negative effects to be positive, beneficial effects. Being high, euphoric, and/or drowsy can, in fact, be pleasant distractions from being a cancer patient.[14] When you have a severe debilitating illness like cancer, feeling high is often an important component of improved well-being, and therefore quality of life.

As my colleague Michelle Sexton and I explained in our recently published journal article, cannabis can enhance feelings of well-being and allow the users to dissociate themselves from their physical symptoms.[15] In fact, medical marijuana is often the only tool that gives cancer patients the lift they so desperately need. Unfortunately, because not all states have legalized medical marijuana, many cancer patients have no other option but to use conventional meds, or perhaps pharmaceutical cannabis if it falls within their doctor's purview.

In addition to favoring cannabis over conventional antiemetics, most cancer patients who use it prefer plant-based rather than prescription synthetic cannabis.[16] And most clinical studies on the effects of cannabis on CINV look at pharmaceuticals that contain only THC. There have, however, been several studies that have evaluated smoked marijuana—which contains both THC and CBD—and concluded that smoking pot was beneficial for relieving nausea and vomiting.[17,18] According to the National Academies of Sciences:

> *[I]t does make sense that inhaling THC in the form of smoked marijuana would prevent vomiting better than swallowing a pill. If vomiting were severe or began immediately after chemotherapy,*

> *oral THC could not stay down long enough to take effect. Smoking also allows patients to take only the drug they want, one puff at a time, thus reducing their risk of unwanted side effects.*[19]

Thus, smoking or vaping cannabis can be helpful because it bypasses the digestive tract and works quickly.[20] There's also abundant anecdotal evidence from both patients and oncologists that inhaled marijuana works well for nausea and vomiting. That said, the risks and benefits of inhaling have to be very carefully weighed.

Smoking and vaping can cause respiratory problems, especially chronic coughing and bronchitis. Recent reports link illegally sold cannabis mixed with vitamin E acetate to an epidemic of the respiratory illness EVALI (e-cigarette or vaping product use-associated lung injury; see Chapter 3). Even if vaping products are sold in reputable dispensaries, it pays to be cautious by carefully checking the ingredients.

A 2020 American Heart Association report on the negative cardiovascular effects of inhaled cannabis recommends that people not smoke or vape cannabis because it can damage the heart, blood vessels, and lungs.[21] These warnings in the era of the COVID-19 pandemic have given my colleagues and me pause about recommending smoking or vaping, especially for cancer patients who are already at high risk, many of whom are older adults—another serious risk factor for COVID.

LOSS OF APPETITE

Loss of appetite (aka anorexia) is extremely common in cancer patients undergoing chemotherapy. Not surprisingly, loss of appetite often goes hand in hand with nausea and vomiting. It's a vicious cycle: if you have no appetite, the thought of food makes you feel nauseated. And if you feel nauseated, you lose your appetite and avoid eating, which can have serious consequences for cancer patients.

They may become undernourished and underweight, putting them at increased risk for infections and other diseases.

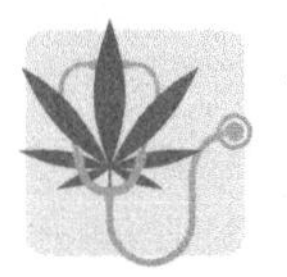

Sophia was lucky that she lived in a state that has legalized medical marijuana and was able to get a recommendation from her doctor. But he told her he didn't know anything about the drug—that she should get information from the dispensary. She did get some useful information and found that smoking or vaping a combination of THC and CBD helped the most. However, she explained, "I brought in chocolate edibles and nibbled a little bit at a time during my chemo sessions because I wasn't allowed to smoke or vape in the treatment room." When she got home, she freely smoked THC and CBD and sometimes ate THC gummy bears. But Sophia often felt terrible for days or even weeks after her treatments; she was very anxious, tired, and had no appetite. "It's not that I was nauseous," she explained. "It was that the thought of eating was nauseating! The smell of food was disgusting and that would make me feel nauseous. Everything has a highly chemical taste. Everything you put in your mouth tastes like poison. I smoked pot and ate gummies for my appetite. I had to eat something! I went from 140 pounds to 115 pounds!"

It's been known for ages that marijuana helps improve appetite (think "the munchies"). Indeed, increasing appetite is one of the top reasons that cancer patients use medical marijuana.[22]

Marijuana munchies is not just a stoner myth; in fact, cannabis is the *only* antiemetic that also increases appetite and even makes eating food more pleasurable,[23] all of which can be highly beneficial for people undergoing chemotherapy. Although there have been very few clinical studies on cannabis as an appetite stimulant in cancer patients, studies involving HIV/AIDS patients, some dating back to the early 2000s, have demonstrated that both smoked pot and Rx cannabis pills can help increase appetite and may help patients gain or maintain weight.[24] A small Canadian study on the effects of pharmaceutical THC on appetite loss and taste changes in advanced cancer patients found that the overwhelming majority reported that their appetites improved significantly and that their food tasted better.[25]

Cancer-related changes in how food tastes and smells are extremely common, affecting almost 90 percent of cancer patients.[26] So even for those who have a good appetite, their once favorite foods may taste and/or smell so terrible they can trigger nausea and vomiting—another vicious cycle. What used to be enjoyable meals with friends or family may become dreaded or even avoided. This is yet another blow to a patient's quality of life that smoking a little weed may help. In addition to giving cancer patients the munchies, weed can enhance the taste of their food and add to their dining pleasure.

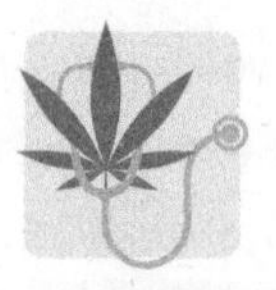

At her cousin's suggestion, Sophia consulted me about her queasiness, loss of appetite, and anxiety. I recommended that she vape pure THC rather than smoke it. In addition to vaping, I suggested she use sublingual 1:1 THC:CBD full-spectrum oil drops with a predominance of calming terpenes (see Chapter 2). I also suggested that she avoid edibles. While they can have a longer and more potent effect, they also can cause more side effects, such as anxiety and fatigue. Taking any type of meds orally isn't a great idea when someone is nauseated or vomits frequently. Sophia said my suggestions worked extremely well; she felt less anxious and had more energy. She was especially pleased that she had never vomited. Although most foods still tasted terrible, her appetite improved. "If I didn't use marijuana to increase my appetite," she explained, "I'd probably weigh under one hundred pounds and be half dead!" She also found that ginger helped a lot. "I craved triple ginger cookies and dark chocolate–covered ginger, as well as Thai food, curries, and anything with turmeric in it, especially ginger tea with turmeric."

Integrative approaches can be very helpful in combating the side effects of cancer treatment, and most cancer patients use them. Table 8-1 below includes the strategies that work especially well for CINV and appetite problems.

TABLE 8-1: INTEGRATIVE APPROACHES FOR NAUSEA AND VOMITING AND LOSS OF APPETITE[27]

NAUSEA & VOMITING	Ginger Acupuncture, acupressure Music therapy Guided imagery therapy
LOSS OF APPETITE & WEIGHT	L-carnitine Melatonin Vitamin E + omega-3 fatty acids Vitamin D Acupuncture

Dr. Kogan's Cannabis Recommendations for Nausea, Vomiting, and Loss of Appetite

In general, when it comes to cancer-related symptoms, THC is a very important player. For CINV and eating problems, I recommend sublingual FECO (full-extract cannabis oil) that is predominantly THC (see Chapter 2). It not only works well, but the effects last longer than inhaled forms. Unless you're very used to taking THC, I suggest starting with 1 to 3 mg and increase each dose slowly until your symptoms are controlled. However, if the nausea and vomiting are severe, increase the THC more quickly—by 1 mg after each dose—and stop increasing when your symptoms are under control. Whether your symptoms are mild or severe, follow my mantra "Stop when you get to where you need to go."

If you prefer vaping, I recommend full-spectrum cannabis extracts or flowers that also are predominantly THC. Just try one or two quick inhales to assess the effect; that's often all that's needed to control nausea for up to several hours. As with sublinguals, you should bump up each dose until the symptoms are controlled.

In addition, I highly recommend that cancer patients take 15 to 30 mg of CBD sublingually twice daily. CBD curbs THC side effects as well as helps relieve anxiety and improve sleep. It also decreases the risk of developing chemotherapy-induced peripheral neuropathy (CIPN), which is discussed later in this chapter. High doses of CBD, especially more than 100 mg a day, should be used with caution because of possible negative interactions with chemotherapy and other medications. Also, although uncommon, some of my older patients who used high doses of CBD at bedtime experienced anxiety. Taking CBD sublingually at lower doses is a much better option. Edible CBD is not a good choice, since its bioavailability (the amount that reaches the bloodstream) is 20 percent or less than the sublingual form.

Another potentially useful but often under-recommended treatment for nausea is the topical application directly over the stomach of THC cream mixed with ginger and cayenne pepper extract. Although this combination may be difficult to find, it's easy to make your own (see Appendix II: Cannabis Resources).

Lastly, rectal suppositories can also work well for CINV and loss of appetite. Although the maximum effect may take more than an hour to kick in, they're good for steady control because the effects are quite long-lasting. I recommend using a 10 to 25 mg THC suppository twice daily. If needed, sublingual or inhaled THC can help with breakthrough nausea.

Although cannabis is an appetite stimulant, increasing appetite in cancer patients is rather unpredictable. Most patients prefer inhaled cannabis to enhance their appetites, although some find that sublingual or edible forms are also effective, so long as they don't induce nausea. CBG (cannabigerol) has recently attracted significant interest. It's a nonintoxicating cannabinoid that has been shown to improve appetite as well as reduce pain and inflammation. (See Chapter 2.) As an extra bonus, animal studies have shown that it can inhibit the growth of certain cancers.[28]

At present, I'm starting to conduct research using CBG as an appetite stimulant. Like CBD, CBG can be derived from hemp, making it easy for patients to obtain in states where medical cannabis is illegal. In fact, CBD:CBG mixtures may be easier to find than pure CBG. A typical starting dose is 5 to 10 mg twice daily, which you can safely increase if necessary. Additionally, some of my cancer patients have reported that CBG has been helpful in relieving their nausea. There's also growing evidence that not only is CBG a potent anti-inflammatory and analgesic, it may even have anticancer effects.[29]

CANCER-RELATED PAIN

Pain is the number one reason cancer patients use medical marijuana. No wonder: pain can severely affect or even destroy a patient's quality of life. And it can strike before, during, and/or after treatment. The pain, which ranges from mild to debilitating, can be caused by the cancer itself, diagnostic tests, cancer treatment, or all of the above. About half of cancer patients suffer from pain at the time of diagnosis.[30] Diagnostic tests, including biopsies, bone marrow aspirations, and endoscopies, among others, can also be extremely painful. Cancer treatment is another culprit, causing pain in more than half of patients undergoing chemotherapy, radiation, and/or surgery,[31] including muscle, joint, and bone pain; painful skin and mouth lesions; and peripheral neuropathy, among others.

Peripheral neuropathy is a chronic nerve condition that can cause pain, numbness, tingling, burning, muscle weakness, and sensitivity to touch and temperature, usually in the feet and legs. It affects about one-third of chemo patients.[32] And chemotherapy-induced peripheral neuropathy (CIPN) is not only one of the most common and debilitating pain problems that afflict cancer patients, it's also one of the most difficult to treat.

Lymphedema, which can be quite painful, is a chronic condition that affects about 16 percent of cancer patients, most of whom have undergone surgery or radiation; however, more than 70 percent of women with breast or gynecological cancer develop this condition after surgery or radiation.[33] These treatments can damage or block the lymph system, causing a buildup of fluid, which most often results in painful swelling of the arms and legs.

Unfortunately, cancer survivors aren't necessarily out of the woods when it comes to pain. For as many as two out of three survivors, lymphedema, peripheral neuropathy, and other painful conditions can persist or occur for the first time months or even years after treatment.[34] Cancer survivors also commonly suffer from sleeping disorders, anxiety, and other psychosocial problems.[35]

Conventional Treatment for Cancer Pain

Most guidelines for treating cancer pain recommend starting with acetaminophen (Tylenol) or non-steroidal anti-inflammatories (NSAIDs), such as aspirin, ibuprofen (Advil), or naproxen (Aleve). These drugs can often be helpful for mild pain, but not for the more serious pain that often afflicts cancer patients. In addition to potentially serious side effects such as kidney and liver damage, these drugs can mask fevers, which makes it difficult for patients undergoing chemo to monitor for infections.

When painkillers don't do the trick, opioids are usually recommended. In fact, opioids are considered the first-line approach for moderate to severe cancer pain management.[36] But they, of course, come with their own set of problems, especially addiction and overdoses, though these are the least common opioid side effects in cancer patients; constipation, drowsiness, nausea, and vomiting occur much more frequently.[37]

Unfortunately, conventional pain remedies—including opioids—often fail to give patients the relief they need. Indeed, it's estimated that as many as half of cancer patients are undertreated for pain because they haven't received the right pain medication or dosage.[38] For example, physicians may under-prescribe opioids because of their side effects or the fear that their patients may become addicted or overdose. Cannabis, by contrast, is nonaddicting and has fewer side effects than opioids and other painkillers. In fact, according to the National Cancer Institute Physician Data Query website, "lethal overdoses from Cannabis and cannabinoids do not occur."[39] Still, some doctors who readily prescribe opioids are hesitant to recommend any form of cannabis to their patients, or they may not even have cannabis on their radar.

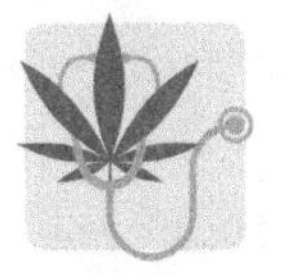

To maximize her chances of survival, Sophia also had a mastectomy. When she left the hospital, her surgeon gave her a prescription for a narcotic painkiller. Sophia told her doctor, "I don't need it; I can get rid of the pain myself with medical marijuana." But her doctor was adamant and said, "You don't understand how serious this is. You'll be in terrible pain!" Sophia promised to fill the prescription and took one pill when she got home. "It made me nauseous and I didn't take another. I vaped a lot of marijuana and ate some gummies." Although she had some discomfort, the cannabis mostly did the trick for her.

Pharmaceutical Cannabinoids for Cancer Pain

While dronabinol (Marinol) and nabilone (Cesamet), the two synthetic THC prescription medications that we described above, have been FDA approved for cancer-related nausea and vomiting, they're rarely recommended or even studied for cancer-related pain. And the few studies that do exist have had mixed results. Still, some recent review articles have concluded that cannabis can be effective in treating neuropathic and/or other chronic pain in cancer patients.[40]

A fairly new and promising pharmaceutical drug, Sativex (nabiximols), is a plant-derived combination of THC and CBD at 1:1 ratio that's been used successfully for the spasticity of multiple sclerosis (see Chapter 9). It has also been found effective for intractable cancer pain, including peripheral neuropathy.[41] Sativex is available in Canada, the United Kingdom, Australia, and many other countries, but because it hasn't been FDA approved, it's not yet available in the United States.

Cannabis for Cancer Pain

Even though cannabis is not yet part of the standard treatment protocol for cancer pain, it's the number one reason cancer patients use pot. This is not surprising, given that both THC and CBD have analgesic effects (see Chapter 2). THC, however, plays a larger role in pain control.

In fact, the ability of marijuana to kill pain—including cancer pain—has been known throughout history. As mentioned in Chapter 1, cannabis was used in ancient China for anesthesia during surgery, and remnants of cannabis were recently found in a 2,500-year-old Siberian burial site of the so-called Siberian Ice Princess, who—according to MRI imaging—had metastatic breast cancer. It's assumed that she used the marijuana to treat her cancer-related pain.[42]

More currently, studies have evaluated smoked or vaped plant-based marijuana on peripheral neuropathy, albeit in non-cancer patients. The studies demonstrated that, even at low doses, marijuana could help treat neuropathic pain.[43] Given the positive results of these studies, it's likely that natural, plant-based pot can also be helpful for patients suffering from CIPN as well as from other cancer-related pain.[44] In fact, a recent study compared the symptoms of cancer patients who used medical marijuana with those who didn't. It looked at their opioid use and ESAS (Edmonton Symptom Assessment System) scores, which measure emotional and physical symptoms, and the authors found that cancer patients who used medical marijuana reduced their use of opioids and had better ESAS scores than non-users.[45] Numerous cancer patient surveys and anecdotal evidence from patients and physicians alike also reaffirm that medical marijuana can help reduce cancer pain.

Unfortunately, as we've explained throughout this book, actual clinical studies on the effects of medical marijuana on cancer and other patients are few and far between. The good news is that this appears to be changing. In a review article my colleagues and I published in 2020, we reported that more clinical trials involving cancer patients are being conducted, and many more are studying natural cannabis.[46] Hopefully, as regulations loosen up, more clinical studies will be conducted on natural, plant-based cannabis and cancer-related pain and other symptoms. Such studies can help shed light on how medical marijuana can help cancer patients.

In addition to being highly effective in killing pain, cannabis also appears to have a "synergistic effect"; it enhances analgesic effects when combined with other painkillers, including opioids.[47] And as mentioned above, cannabis not only helps reduce patients' pain when used along with opioids but can also help these patients cut down on their opioid doses.[48] (See Chapter 4.) In fact, there's increasing evidence that cannabis can help cancer patients quit using opioids and other painkillers altogether.[49] This substitution effect is also seen in other pain patients who use pot (see Chapters 4 and 5).

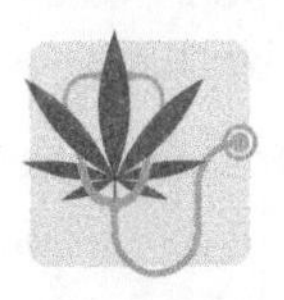

At seventy-two, Ben, a retired teacher, was diagnosed with moderately advanced prostate cancer, which was successfully treated with a combination of hormonal therapy and radiation. However, he continued to have a lot

of disturbing symptoms, including severe pain when urinating and frequent anxiety. Ben also lost his appetite and as a result lost a lot of weight. He was prescribed a lot of painkillers, including oxycodone and other opioids, but they didn't work particularly well. When he came to see me, I recommended that he use rectal cannabis THC suppositories and occasionally try THC-infused edibles. He also did pelvic floor physical therapy exercises to help relieve pelvic floor muscle spasms and painful urination. This combination treatment helped improve Ben's appetite; he gained ten pounds and became considerably less anxious. But most important, within a few weeks his pain was almost completely gone. After about six months Ben was able to gradually decrease his use of suppositories and has since remained pain-free. He continues to occasionally use sublingual drops and edibles 1:1 THC:CBD to relieve anxiety and help him sleep. I see Ben frequently, and now, years later, he's still doing well and is no longer having pelvic pain.

Dr. Kogan's Cannabis Recommendations for Cancer-Related Pain

Unfortunately, pain caused by cancer is difficult to treat and usually requires high doses of cannabis, sometimes with different routes of delivery, such as topicals, sublinguals, or suppositories. Treating the pain depends on the type of cancer and the type of pain. In general, I believe it's best to deliver cannabis close to the source of pain. For example, I've had several male patients with prostate cancer that metastasized to the lower back who did well with rectal suppositories of 10 to 25 mg of THC. Some patients find that adding CBD helps. According to a recent Israeli study of medical marijuana use in cancer survivors, most of the survivors (90 percent) used marijuana for pain relief.[50] (Sleeping problems and anxiety came in second and third.)

The majority preferred smoking pot, usually with either equal ratios of THC and CBD or higher levels of CBD. Others preferred vaping or topical applications.

Patients with severe pain often find relief from combining cannabis with opioids or other painkillers. The good news is that not only is this combination safe, it appears to be safer and more effective than taking a large dose of opioids alone.[51] As discussed above, this synergistic effect often helps these patients reduce or even quit their use of opioids.

For my patients with chemotherapy-induced peripheral neuropathy, I recommend two steps. The first is a preventive measure for patients undergoing chemo with drugs known to cause CIPN. This involves starting on a low dose of CBD (15 to 50 mg) sublingually twice a day before or during chemo. The second step involves treatment of the symptoms with a triple or quadruple topical application of 1:1:1 THC:CBD:CBDa or 1:1:1:1 THC:CBD:THCa:CBDa. As explained in Chapter 3, CBDa has a strong effect similar to that of NSAIDs such as ibuprofen and naproxen; it reduces inflammation and thus helps relieve pain. If this triple or quadruple topical is not available, then I recommend trying a 1:1 THC:CBD cream. It's also a good idea to add capsaicin (pharmaceutical-grade cayenne pepper) to the cream. This can act synergistically, increasing the effectiveness of the topical treatment (see Chapter 3).

If topicals fail to work, I recommend trying sublingual or inhaled cannabis. In general, the cannabis dose needed to control CIPN doesn't have to be very high. I find that for sublingual or inhaled cannabis, most patients do well with 2 to 5 mg of THC several times a day. For sublinguals, I usually suggest a 1:1 THC:CBD or THC-predominant FECO oil, starting with 2 to 3 mg of THC and increasing it slowly until you find relief. Follow my marijuana mantra: "Go slow until you get to where you need to go!" If their CIPN is worse at night—unfortunately an all-too-common occurrence—edibles or other oral forms of THC may help because their effects can last longer than other methods of delivery. Most people find starting out with 5 mg of a THC-infused edible is a reasonable place to begin. However, if you're an experienced pot user, you can start with a higher dose of THC, but be sure to increase your dose very slowly.

I'm often asked if CIPN—which is considered a lifelong condition—can be curable. In my practice, I've seen several cases of CIPN completely cured. These patients have used a combination of the cannabinoids mentioned above, high-dose nutrients, and acupuncture. Even if a total cure isn't achieved, this combination can help relieve symptoms in many patients, even in some of the most severe cases.

TABLE 8-2: INTEGRATIVE APPROACHES FOR PERIPHERAL NEUROPATHY[52]

Chemotherapy-induced peripheral neuropathy (CIPN)	B-vitamins Acupuncture Vitamin E L-glutamine Omega-3 fatty acids

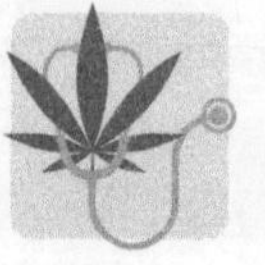

Mary, a seventy-five-year-old piano teacher, was diagnosed with pancreatic cancer. She underwent chemotherapy, but the tumor invaded a large nerve near her pancreas and was causing severe pain. Surgery was out of the question, and opiates not only didn't work, but they also caused severe constipation and nausea. Although a nerve block worked well initially, the effects didn't last very long. Mary finally got relief from a combination of 25 mg of THC suppositories and gummies (4:1 CBD:THC ratio). In addition, Mary occasionally used sublingual drops of cannabis to control nausea and enhance her appetite.

Cancer patients tend to have many different symptoms, and no one treatment can address them all. But cannabis comes close; no other single treatment can help relieve pain, reduce anxiety, improve sleep, increase appetite, decrease nausea and vomiting, and even improve quality of life.

QUALITY OF LIFE

The importance of improving quality of life can't be overstated. That's where euphoria comes in. Although euphoria is usually listed as an adverse side effect of marijuana, it's often one of the most important therapeutic benefits for very sick patients. If marijuana causes patients to feel euphoric, high, or even stoned, and gives them respite from their medical reality, it's good medicine . . . not an adverse effect. As my colleague Dr. Donald Abrams, a world-renowned cannabis expert and oncologist, poignantly put it: "I ask all of my patients, 'What brings you joy?' The number of cancer patients who answer 'gardening' is not insignificant. I think if you feel that part of you has died or you are dying, the ability to bring life out of the ground is a blessing. And if you can grow your own medicine, that is very empowering!"

Dr. S. K. Aggarwal, one of the top experts in the use of cannabis in palliative care (see Chapter 9), agrees:

> *A mild euphoria or sense of well-being, if brought about through use of cannabinoid botanical products, could very well play an important therapeutic role for patients faced with the despair of a terminal malady and the loss of function that normally accompanies it.*[53]

This topic often touches me at the core of my being. I can give you a sense of the power cannabis has for alleviating suffering at the end of life by relating the story of one of my patients, Norma, who recently passed away from metastatic breast cancer. Norma was not dying easily. When I first met her, she was undergoing cancer care at a top academic center, but she still suffered from severe abdominal pain and couldn't eat because she vomited up most of her food. She also suffered from severe anxiety and panic attacks. As often happens in such situations, most of my interactions were with her family. With their consent, I introduced cannabis into her care. It had a major positive impact on Norma's last days, which actually became last weeks and last months. Norma's daughter wrote to me that she died peacefully, surrounded by her loving family.

Dealing with dying patients can be an emotionally painful process for family members. But it's also hard on the medical staff as well. Now, many months after Norma died, when I'm having a hard time dealing with these challenging situations, I need to remind myself why I'm doing what I'm doing, and that it can make an enormous difference to patients and their families. I sometimes reread Norma's daughter's message to me the morning after her mother passed away.

> *I am writing to express my immense gratitude for all you did for my beloved and precious mother these last six months. She passed away last night around 7:40 p.m. Thanks to you, with all her meds, she remained pain-free and nausea-free. Later when anxiety took over, you provided wonderful solutions for that as well. At last, her long and valiant struggle has ended. Thank you for being there for her and for us and for your compassionate and timely counsel through this journey.*

I'm gratified that the medical cannabis may have helped prolong Norma's life by treating her symptoms and improving her quality of life. Unfortunately, cannabis couldn't cure her breast cancer.

CAN CANNABIS CURE CANCER?

While there's abundant medical evidence that cannabis can be immensely helpful in treating cancer symptoms and side effects, there is absolutely no evidence that it can cure cancer. Unfortunately, there's a plethora of misinformation about the benefits of marijuana for curing cancer. This is a highly emotional and controversial topic, and we want to be totally clear: *we do not in any way advocate the use of cannabis as a substitute for conventional cancer treatments*, which have been proven to successfully treat or stop the spread of many cancers. And there is *no* clinical evidence that cannabis treatment alone can cure cancer. To the contrary, as my coauthors and I warned in our recently published journal article, refusing conventional cancer treatment in favor of medical marijuana (or other complementary treatments) can reduce the chances of a patient's survival.[54]

While the notion that smoking pot can cure cancer may be just a pipe dream, it's a dream that might not entirely go up in smoke. Since 1975, numerous lab studies have demonstrated that THC and CBD could induce "autophagy"—a process by which cancer cells "eat" themselves—as well as "apoptosis"—a process by which cancer cells can kill themselves.[55]

Recent lab studies on animal and human cells have confirmed these findings; they've demonstrated that THC, CBD, and other cannabinoids can both prevent cancer cells from growing and spreading

---

CANNABIS QUOTE

"One of the more distressing situations that oncologists increasingly face is trying to counsel the patient who has a curable diagnosis, but who seeks to forgo conventional cancer treatment in favor of depending on cannabis oil to eradicate their malignancy because of the large number of online testimonials from people claiming such results. Given my long practice in San Francisco, I can assume that a large proportion of my patients have used cannabis during their journey. If cannabis cured cancer, I would have a lot more survivors in my practice today."

—Donald I. Abrams, MD, oncologist and cannabis specialist[56]

---

and can actually kill the cancer cells. A review article was just published about the potential benefits of cannabinoids for melanoma, the deadliest form of skin cancer. Although most of the studies they reviewed were conducted on animals, the authors concluded that cannabinoids not only were able to kill melanoma cancer cells but helped prevent the cancer cells from spreading.[57] According to the authors, cannabis extracts, although not a cure, do "have the potential not only to enhance survival rates but also to potentially improve the quality of life in melanoma patients."[58]

There have also been a few small clinical studies on patients being treated for glioblastoma, a very serious brain cancer, that have had positive results. Depending on the study, patients were given synthetic THC or THC/CBD (Sativex) in addition to chemotherapy.[59] Even though clinical studies are limited, it does appear that the combination of cannabis and chemo may help prolong the patients' lives.[60]

Because of the difficulties of conducting any clinical trials using THC, we're not expecting the anticancer benefits of cannabis proven or disproven in clinical settings anytime soon. This puts patients who have cancer now in a dilemma. While scientific and clinical data is lacking, the internet is full of often false claims of cannabis cures, and more and more patients are trying different forms, often at their peril.

In addition to anecdotal evidence from patients (that may or may not be true), I and other physicians who work with cancer patients and cannabis are seeing occasional cases that appear to be too good to be true. Some of the most striking cancer cure cases I have seen in my practice have involved cannabis being used along with conventional cancer treatment.

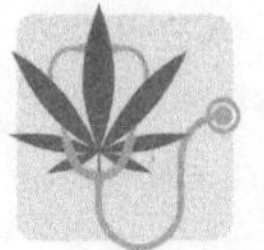

Harry, a sixty-year-old florist, had stage IV aggressive colon cancer. He was told that even with chemotherapy and surgery, his life expectancy was only six to ten months. When I first saw him, he had decided to start chemotherapy and was already using Rick Simpson Oil (RSO), a high-

dose THC formula that has been touted as a cancer cure. He told me that he also wanted to try some integrative approaches and went on a high-fat, low-carb vegetarian diet. In addition, he took fish oil and probiotics, and was having intravenous vitamin C infusions. After he finished three rounds of chemo, Harry underwent "debulking" surgery, a palliative procedure that decreases the number of tumors but doesn't cure the cancer. When they opened him up, there was no sign of cancer! The surgeon said to me, "I have never seen anything like this in my entire twenty-five-plus years of experience!" My colleagues and I have since reported this case at a recent medical conference.[61]

It's not clear whether it was the cannabis, the other approaches, or a combination that was responsible for Harry's "miracle cure." As we mentioned above, there's increasing evidence that various forms of cannabis, when used in conjunction with conventional chemotherapy and/or radiation, can help these treatments become more successful and increase the chances of remission.[62]

Cannabis terpenes also have a key role to play in cancer prevention and treatment. In addition to being responsible for the aroma and flavor of cannabis, terpenes have many proven health benefits, such as helping reduce anxiety, depression, and pain, to name a few (see Chapter 2). According to a recent review article, lab and animal studies have also demonstrated that some terpenes have the ability to help kill certain cancer cells.[63] For example, β-caryophyllene was found to have anticancer effects in lung, ovarian, and skin cancers. And linalool and pinene appear to help treat some skin cancers as well as possibly prevent them. Limonene has anti–breast and –oral cancer effects. And although myrcene has caused some cancers in mice and rats, it appears to help kill cervical, lung, and colon cancer cells.

In addition, according to a recent review article, cannabinoids—especially CBD—have been shown to act synergistically with chemotherapy and/or radiation to increase the effectiveness of cancer treatments.[64]

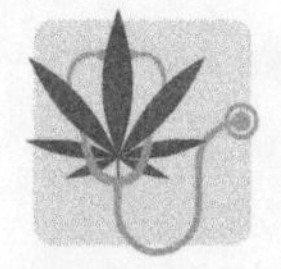

Sophia—the jewelry designer with stage IV metastatic breast cancer—initially used medical marijuana for the side effects of the strong chemotherapy she received. The pot worked extremely well in controlling her nausea, post-mastectomy pain, and other side effects. It also helped relieve her anxiety and lift her mood. And it appears that there was an added bonus; after one year of treatment, Sophia was told that she was cancer-free! Such a "cure" (which her oncologist insisted on calling it, rather than a "remission") is extremely rare. She attributes her "cure" not only to the aggressive treatment she received, but to medical marijuana, which she continues to use to this day. She believes it will help reduce the chances of a recurrence.

So while there's no proof that cannabis can directly cure cancer, there is reason to be optimistic. And if one day cannabis will be shown to be effective for treating cancer, I believe that the daily doses would have to be very high, around 1000 mg of total cannabinoids. The doses would also be a complex mix of FECOs with different ratios of THC, THCa, CBD, CBDa, and CBG, which could be administered orally, sublingually, and rectally.

Cannabis, terpenes, and cancer treatment can all work together to vastly improve the survival of cancer patients. While cannabis may be helpful in treating some cancers, it should *only* be used along with conventional cancer treatment to manage cancer-related symptoms. Medical marijuana may not be the magic bullet that can cure cancer. However, it's still one of the best drugs in our arsenal to alleviate the terrible effects of cancer and cancer treatment and help improve the quality of life for millions of patients, and hopefully prolong those lives as well.

CHAPTER NINE

Chronic Neurological Conditions

Chronic neurological disorders are among the most challenging to treat and—more important—difficult to live with. People with such conditions as multiple sclerosis (MS), Parkinson's disease (PD), and Alzheimer's disease (AD) may have trouble with their motor control, cognition, mood, and memory, all of which can drastically affect the quality of their lives.

The discovery in 2014 that CBD can reduce epileptic seizures, followed in 2018 by the FDA's approval of the plant-derived CBD drug Epidiolex (cannabidiol), was a game changer for people who suffer from epilepsy and other seizure disorders. This breakthrough has been good news for the millions of sufferers of other chronic neurological conditions; it has spurred interest in researching the benefits of CBD and THC. The benefits of cannabis for the spasticity and pain of MS are already well documented. And there's now increasing evidence that medical marijuana can be beneficial for many of the other disturbing and debilitating symptoms of MS, as well as those of Parkinson's and Alzheimer's diseases.

MULTIPLE SCLEROSIS (MS)

MS, a chronic, degenerative disease of the central nervous system, affects about a million people in the United States. It usually strikes between the ages of twenty and forty, and women are about three times more likely than men to develop it. Common symptoms include pain, spasticity, insomnia, fatigue, bladder and bowel problems, walking difficulties, depression, cognitive decline, and vision changes. The symptoms, which usually start out slowly, progress over time and can severely interfere with day-to-day functioning and quality of life. Unfortunately, MS is not curable, and although there are myriad medical treatments available, the symptoms are very difficult to control.

Conventional Treatments for MS

Because MS is currently incurable, treatment focuses on relieving symptoms, preventing and managing flare-ups, and slowing the progression of the disease. Corticosteroids, such as prednisone, are commonly prescribed and can help control some of the symptoms. But they can have disturbing side effects, including fluid retention, weight gain, high blood pressure, insomnia, mood changes, and increased risk of infections. For more severe cases and flare-ups, stronger so-called disease-modifying drugs—such as interferon—may be prescribed. These drugs—which affect the immune system—typically involve injections or infusions and can carry even more adverse effects and risks, including fever, infections, and liver damage. Plus, they can cost more than $70,000 a year![1]

Cannabis Treatment for MS

Given that conventional treatments aren't especially helpful, that their side effects can sometimes be worse than the MS symptoms, and that the costs may be sky-high, increasing numbers of MS sufferers are understandably turning to medical marijuana.[2] In fact, a recent, large web-based survey conducted by the National Multiple Sclerosis Society (NMSS) and the Michael J. Fox Foundation (MJFF) found that 66 percent of MS patients who responded to the survey were currently using marijuana for symptom relief.[3] In addition, the overwhelming majority of pot-using patients found it helpful for their MS symptoms, especially spasticity and pain,[4] and research is bearing that out. According to a large review article published in the prestigious *Journal of the American Medical Association* (*JAMA*), "use of marijuana for . . . spasticity due to multiple sclerosis is supported by high-quality evidence."[5]

Most of the cannabis clinical studies on MS used FDA-approved Rx drugs like Cesamet (nabilone) and Marinol (dronabinol), or Sativex (nabiximols), which is not yet FDA approved (see Chapter 2). Even though the studies have demonstrated that they can help relieve pain and spasticity, these drugs are not very popular with MS (and other) patients, primarily because of their unpleasant side effects, which can include dry mouth, drowsiness, dizziness, disorientation, and memory problems, among others.

However, based on the results of these studies, researchers believe that cannabis may be useful for treating the other common MS problems: sleep, mood, and mobility.[6] Although clinical research on the use of cannabis for these specific symptoms is lacking, there's ample anecdotal evidence and surveys that confirm that many MS patients find medical marijuana helpful for these and other problems. For example, one survey found that the majority of marijuana-using MS patients who used pot for pain and sleeping problems reported that these symptoms improved by more than 60 percent.[7] Medical marijuana has also been reported to help relieve tremors, urinary and sexual problems, and vision disturbances.[8] And, according to the NMSS/MJFF study mentioned above, compared with abstainers, pot-using MS patients reported lower levels of disability as measured by mood, memory, and fatigue.[9] In addition, almost 80 percent of those users said they reduced their consumption of prescription drugs. A more recent survey found similarly high rates of MS patients were able to quit or reduce their use of prescription drugs, including opioids, because they found medical cannabis to be more effective.[10] These are other examples of the substitution effect (the preference for cannabis over conventional meds), which is discussed throughout this book.

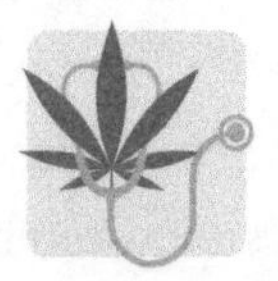

Amy, a forty-one-year-old project manager for a nonprofit organization in Virginia, had MS. Although she wasn't bothered by pain or spasticity, the MS was severely affecting her vision. She decided to make major lifestyle changes, including switching to an organic vegan diet and taking a high dose of vitamin D, all of which helped resolve her vision problem. However, she still didn't feel up to par. She had heard that medical marijuana can be helpful for MS symptoms, but it wasn't legal in Virginia at the time. I recommended that she try sublingual CBD oil starting with 12.5 mg twice daily and slowly titrating up. She described the CBD as "a godsend." Not only did Amy feel much better physically, her alertness and ability to concentrate were dramatically improved. She said that she hadn't realized until she took CBD just how much the MS affected her ability to think clearly. Amy has since started a blog on the benefits of CBD for MS.

Dr. Kogan's Cannabis Recommendations for MS

Most of the studies supporting marijuana use in MS have been conducted on patients who primarily use the inhaled route of administration. The majority of my MS patients prefer smoking or vaping, mostly because they have a rapid onset of action. Although I think the inhaled route may be a reasonable choice to control the symptoms of MS for some, I believe that the sublingual route is better, as well as safer, especially in light of COVID (see Chapter 3). In fact, quite a few of my patients with MS tell me that they feel symptomatically better with sublingual FECO (full-extract cannabis oil)—my favorite form of medical cannabis for MS and many other conditions (see Chapter 2)—than they do when they smoke. For someone with early MS, I suggest starting with sublingual FECO that has 1 to 2 mg THC and a high ratio of CBD (5:1 to 10:1 THC:CBD). Ideally, it would also contain CBDa, and possibly THCa and CBG, all of which are described in Chapter 2. And my marijuana mantra "Start low, go slow" definitely applies.

While I hear lots of claims that pure CBD can help "cure" MS and other neurodegenerative diseases, I haven't found this to be true in my practice. It's possible that very high doses of CBD (1000 mg/day), which is available as a prescription drug (Epidiolex), might someday be proven to be effective in treating MS. But I can't advocate for it now because of the lack of evidence and high cost, which can be thousands of dollars per month. In addition, because many patients with MS and other neurological conditions take a number of other medications, there's a real possibility of negative drug interactions with high doses of CBD.

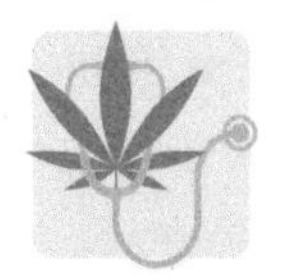

In the early 1960s, when Jules was in his thirties, he was diagnosed with multiple sclerosis. The only thing his doctors could offer him was the suggestion that he move to a warmer climate. Jules, his wife, Libby, and their two

children, Stephanie and Mark, moved from DC to Miami, where the heat and humidity only made his pain, spasms, and other MS symptoms worse. His Miami doctor prescribed a number of drugs that didn't help, including steroids and Talwin, an opioid that was supposed to be nonaddicting but has since been withdrawn from the market. In fact, Jules wound up addicted to Talwin and had to go into the hospital to detox. Another doctor suggested he try marijuana, even though it was illegal. Jules, a straitlaced businessman with young children at home, was hesitant. But out of desperation, he decided to try pot, which he smoked in joints or in a pipe. Jules finally found a treatment, albeit an illegal one, that relieved not only his peripheral neuropathies and muscle spasms but his anxiety and depression as well. Luckily, he was able to get it from some sympathetic health aides who were aware of the medical benefits. Without their help, his symptoms would have been much worse. He and Libby later moved to New Jersey, where other sympathetic aides were able to get him the only drug that helped his MS symptoms.

In 2005, Jules died at age seventy-five of unrelated causes, and four years later, Libby was diagnosed with lung cancer. She was treated with chemotherapy and lost her appetite and forty-five pounds. Her doctors recommended marijuana, but she couldn't find it because it was still illegal. Unfortunately, she died two months later. Their daughter, Stephanie, a public health nurse in DC, was so outraged that her parents had to struggle to find marijuana for their debilitating diseases that she decided to do something about it. When medical cannabis became legal in DC, in 2010, she and her husband, Jeffrey, a retired rabbi, decided to open a dispensary, and asked me to help them with the medical and practical aspects of the business. In 2013, Stephanie and Jeffrey opened the Tacoma Wellness Center, the first medical cannabis dispensary in the DC area, the walls of which are graced with photos of Jules and Libby.

PARKINSON'S DISEASE (PD)

Parkinson's disease is a degenerative movement disorder that affects 1 million people in the United States, most of whom are men over the age of sixty. Although the exact cause is unknown, it's believed to be the result of a combination of environmental and genetic factors.[11] About 15 percent of Parkinson's patients have a family history of the disease,[12] and it's more prevalent among certain ethnic groups, especially Ashkenazi Jews and North African Arab Berbers.[13] Common symptoms include slow movement (bradykinesia), poor balance and coordination, body stiffness, and resting tremors. Resting tremors are one of the hallmarks of Parkinson's disease. As their name implies, they occur when hands, fingers, arms, or legs are at rest.

As the disease progresses, other symptoms may occur, including sleep problems, depression, trouble speaking, and chewing or swallowing difficulties. People with PD may also suffer from constipation, urinary and sexual problems, difficulty focusing, and hallucinations.

PD symptoms are the result of a deficiency of dopamine, a chemical produced in the brain that controls body movements, emotions, and cognition, among other key functions. There is no specific diagnostic test for PD; rather, diagnosis is based on the symptoms mentioned above. While these symptoms can sometimes be managed by a variety of medications, there is unfortunately no cure yet.

PILL ROLLING

Some people with PD also have a type of resting tremor referred to as "pill rolling." They make uncontrollable circular finger movements that look like they're rolling a pill between their fingers and thumb. Cannabinoids, especially THC, have been shown to help relieve resting and other kinds of tremors.[14]

Conventional Treatment for Parkinson's Disease

Because there are no current treatments available to stop the progression of PD, conventional treatments are aimed at controlling the motor symptoms mentioned above. The gold standard of PD treatment is L-dopa (levodopa), a drug that converts into dopamine when it reaches the brain. Virtually all PD patients are prescribed this drug, which can help control tremors, stiffness, and slow movements. However, while it may provide relief of some motor symptoms, L-dopa does not prevent the progression of PD. Additionally, most people who take L-dopa experience nausea and vomiting. To control these unpleasant side effects, L-dopa is usually combined with another drug, carbidopa. Ironically, while this combination can be very helpful for some PD symptoms, it, too, can cause nausea, as well as low blood pressure and confusion.

Another problem is that L-dopa is only useful during the early or intermediate stages of PD. Its effectiveness diminishes over time and causes patients' symptoms to fluctuate, which is referred to as the "on/off effect." A more serious concern is that after long-term use most patients develop irreversible dyskinesia: involuntary, jerky, or repetitive movements of the face, lips, tongue, arms, or legs.[15]

Some patients are prescribed "dopamine agonists," which mimic the effects of dopamine. Although these drugs may be less likely than L-dopa to cause dyskinesia, they're not as effective for treating motor symptoms. Plus, they, too, can have disturbing side effects, including drowsiness, swollen legs, confusion, and hallucinations, and can trigger compulsive eating, sexual conduct, gambling, and shopping, among other disturbing behaviors.

Conventional treatments also don't address the numerous non-motor symptoms that plague virtually all PD patients.[16] These symptoms, which sometimes occur even before the classic motor symptoms of PD, include pain, trouble sleeping, depression, anxiety, constipation, loss of sense of smell and taste, difficulty swallowing, drooling, urinary problems, cognitive impairment, hallucinations, psychosis, and sexual problems. All of these can take a tremendous toll on a patient's quality of life and can even be more disabling and disturbing than PD's motor symptoms. Unfortunately, these non-motor symptoms are frequently overlooked by physicians who tend to focus on their patients' classic motor symptoms. And patients may be reluctant or embarrassed to discuss these problems with their doctors because they may not realize that they're also symptoms of PD.[17]

Cannabis Treatment for Parkinson's Disease

Given the lack of long-term effectiveness of conventional PD treatments for both motor and non-motor symptoms, as well as their disturbing or even dangerous side effects, it's understandable that most PD patients turn to medical marijuana and other alternative treatments. In fact, according to a recent physician survey, 80 percent of their PD patients used some form of weed for their PD symptoms.[18]

A number of recent journal articles have concluded that patients who smoke or vape weed have reported finding relief from motor

POT IN THE PAST

Cannabis was first mentioned as a treatment for tremors in 1888 by William Gowers, MD, who was considered "the father of British neurology." In his textbook *A Manual of Diseases of the Nervous System*, Gowers wrote that oral extracts of Indian hemp relieved tremors.[19] He also wrote that arsenic, morphine, and hemlock could be effective for tremor control, but added that he found that the combination of Indian hemp and opium was the most effective tremor treatment.[20]

symptoms, including resting tremors, rigidity, and bradykinesia (slow movements).[21] And some small studies and surveys have found that PD patients who smoked pot reported not only improvement in their motor problems but in their sleeping, pain, mood, and quality of life.[22]

One of the largest studies looking at marijuana use in both MS and PD patients was the Michael J. Fox and National Multiple Sclerosis Society survey mentioned above.[23] More than one-third of the 450 PD patients who responded to the survey said they used marijuana. Compared with nonusers, significantly more pot users with PD reported lower levels of disability, especially with regard to mood, memory, and fatigue. And almost half of the users reduced their prescription PD medications—more evidence that the substitution effect is a real phenomenon.

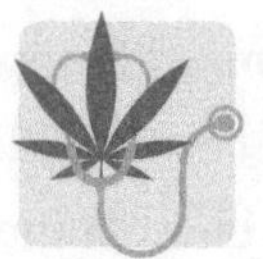

When Tom, a retired college professor, was seventy-five years old, he developed Parkinson's disease. Although he suffered from classic PD symptoms, including tremors, rigidity, fatigue, insomnia, and constipation, he refused to take any conventional medications. His doctor referred him to me for integrative treatment. I first recommended a Mediterranean, anti-inflammatory diet and several supplements, including magnesium, fish oil, and CoQ10. I then recommended that Tom take a FECO mixture of 1:1 THC:CBD sublingually, which totally and quickly resolved his sleeping problems. An additional twice-a-day sublingual dose of FECO that was high in CBD helped improve his concentration. I also suggested that Tom try vaping a high dose of THC for his tremors. Although it helped, the positive effects only lasted for a short period of time. Plus, he didn't like the euphoric effect, which he said interfered with his ability to carry out his daily activities, so he stuck with sublingual THC and CBD.

Dr. Kogan's Cannabis Recommendations for Parkinson's Disease

I see lots of patients with PD in my practice and recommend medical cannabis to many. Cannabis helps these patients manage almost all the common symptoms of the disease, including tremors, rigidity, muscle spasms, nausea, insomnia, and anxiety. My marijuana mantra "Start low, go slow" is especially applicable to PD patients. Many suffer from dizziness, gait imbalances, and lack of coordination, all of which can put them at risk for falls and other accidents. They may also have concentration and memory difficulties. Because the potential side effects of THC include dizziness, visual changes, impaired cognition, and short-term memory loss, people with PD—especially older adults—need to use it with caution. As mentioned above, I prefer most of my patients with neurodegenerative conditions to take sublingual FECO that contains both THC and CBD.

Medical marijuana can do wonders for PD patients, especially those who have trouble sleeping (see Chapter 5). Sleeping problems can be a very serious problem for patients with PD or other chronic neurological conditions because their symptoms worsen considerably when their sleep is disrupted. If they have trouble sleeping, I suggest sublingual FECO at a very low dose of 1 to 3 mg of 1:1 THC:CBD or THC:CBN at bedtime, and to then titrate up slowly. CBN (cannabinol), close cousin to CBD, has mild psychoactive effects (see Chapter 2) and has the most sedative effects of all the cannabinoids. When combined with THC, it is an excellent choice for sleep problems. Once sleep improves, stop increasing the dose. More is not always better; too much marijuana can cause unpleasant side effects without any additional benefits.

Sublingual or oral FECO that is high in THC and made from strains that contain sedating terpenes can also work very well for sleeping problems. The dose of THC should still start low (1 to 3 mg) and slowly be titrated up as needed. Sedating terpenes found in different cannabis strains include β-caryophyllene, limonene, linalool, and myrcene (see Chapter 2). For patients taking high doses of THC, I recommend adding 15 to 30 mg of sublingual CBD twice daily to minimize the risk of side effects of the THC. High doses of oral (edible or capsules) CBD of more than 100 mg should be taken with caution. Too much CBD can interact with other PD medications. That's why sublingual CBD is by far the preferred method; it bypasses the gut and is unlikely to cause negative interactions with other medications. It also has high bioavailability, so less is needed, which lowers the cost.

ALZHEIMER'S DISEASE (AD)

Alzheimer's disease is arguably the most feared disease among older adults. And for good reason: it robs both the elderly and their families of normal lives. This dreadful disease affects about 6 million people in the United States. While Alzheimer's most often strikes people over the age of seventy-five,[24] the majority of patients with this disease are between eighty and eighty-five.[25] Unfortunately, the number of people with AD is expected to rise dramatically in the coming years because of our aging population. Although there are other forms of dementia with similar symptoms, AD is by far the most common.

In the early stages, AD can affect memory, reasoning, and language. As the disease progresses, memory grows worse and confusion sets in. People with AD may no longer recognize family members and friends. They may start to develop behavioral problems and psychotic symptoms, such as hallucinations, delusions, paranoia, and extreme agitation. Agitation often goes hand in hand with aggression and is one of the most distressing and challenging AD symptoms for patients, caregivers, and physicians. Agitation also leads to higher rates of institutionalization and death.[26]

Conventional Treatment for AD

Not only does AD diminish a patient's quality of life, robbing them of their autonomy, it also increases caregivers' burden and stress. Unfortunately, despite decades of research and the more than two hundred drugs that have been developed to treat AD, not a single one has proven very effective in treating AD symptoms or improving quality of life.[27] Even more discouraging is that the FDA has approved only one new drug to treat AD since 2003. And there's no conclusive evidence that this drug, which was approved in 2021, works or is safe. Even when they do help treat some symptoms, the benefits of AD drugs only last about a year. In spite of this, the majority of AD patients are prescribed these drugs for much longer, sometimes up to ten years.[28] These drugs are not only ineffective, they can also have such adverse side effects as nausea, vomiting, diarrhea, fatigue, insomnia, and loss of appetite and weight. And some AD meds can have even more serious side effects—such as slow heart rate, dizziness, and falling—which can lead to hip fractures. Antipsychotics and other drugs commonly used to treat agitation and other common AD behavioral problems can increase the risk of stroke and death.[29] Although these drugs have a "black box warning,"* they're prescribed "off label" to one-third of dementia patients in nursing homes.[30] In addition to their poor effectiveness and potentially serious side effects, none of these AD drugs can slow the progression of the disease, delay institutionalization, or increase survival.[31] Cannabis, on the other hand, appears to be both a more promising and a safer treatment.[32]

---

* Black box warnings are required by the FDA on some prescription drugs to call attention to serious or life-threatening risk.

Cannabis Treatment for AD

The therapeutic benefits of cannabis for MS, PD, and other neurological conditions are attributed to its anti-inflammatory, antioxidant, and neuroprotective effects. Based on these positive effects and the promising results of research studies, there's reason to believe that cannabis can be useful in treating AD as well.[33]

Although the exact cause of Alzheimer's and other dementias is unknown, amyloid plaques (aka "senile plaques") are thought to be a major factor. In fact, the presence of amyloid plaques on brain scans is considered the hallmark of AD. These plaques are made up of "amyloid beta," sticky clumps of protein that destroy brain cells and cause cognitive decline. A recent lab study found that THC not only reduced inflammation but amyloid beta as well.[34] Some studies in mice have demonstrated that a combination of THC and CBD also decreased levels of amyloid beta as well as reversing learning impairments,[35] providing even more evidence that cannabis may play an important role in the treatment of Alzheimer's disease.

There have been only a few clinical studies that have involved cannabis and AD, but they have had promising results. According to a recent review article, several of these studies have reported significant improvement in patients with late-stage AD who were given FDA-approved synthetic THC, dronabinol (Marinol). The patients became less agitated, slept better, and gained weight.[36] The authors concluded that cannabis may decrease some AD symptoms and may actually slow the progression of the disease—something no other drug has been able to do.

One of the most recent and well-designed studies found that those patients who received another synthetic THC, Cesamet (nabilone), had significantly less agitation and were less of a burden to caregivers than those who received a placebo.[37] However, nabilone has potentially serious side effects, including oversedation and cognitive decline. And because it's not usually covered by Medicare, it comes at the high price of $10,000 to $15,000 per month on average.[38]

Unfortunately, only a few studies have involved treating AD patients with natural cannabis. In one of these studies, which was conducted in a California nursing home, patients received cannabis preparations as a tincture or a sweet edible.[39] Not only did the patients' sleep and mood improve, but their agitation, pain, and nursing-care demands also decreased. And in a small Canadian study, when Alzheimer's patients were given MCO (medical cannabis oil) containing 2.5 mg of THC over a period of four weeks, agitation, aggression, delusions, nighttime behavior and sleep problems, and caregiver distress significantly declined.[40]

In a more recent, small pilot study in Switzerland, patients with severe dementia were given increasingly high doses of natural THC/CBD oil over a period of two months.[41] To make the drug more palatable and easier to administer, the cannabis oil was put on small pieces of chocolate cake. After two months, behavior problems, especially screaming, aggression, and tearing off clothes, decreased measurably, and none of the patients experienced significant side effects. Family members reported to the researchers that they were pleased with the results. And the nurses, many of whom were initially very skeptical about using marijuana on AD patients, reported that their patients were more relaxed, less irritable, and smiled more often—all of which helped make nursing care less difficult.

Based on these clinical and preclinical studies, according to a recent review article by world-renowned cannabis researcher Ethan Russo, there's reason to be optimistic that cannabis may be a safe and effective treatment for relieving AD symptoms.[42] The authors of another recent review article concluded the following:

> *[M]edical cannabis may be effective for treating neuropsychiatric symptoms associated with dementia (i.e., agitation, disinhibition, irritability, aberrant motor behaviour, nocturnal behaviour*

disorders, and aberrant vocalization and resting care). There was also limited evidence of improvement in rigidity and cognitive scores.[43]

Dr. Kogan's Cannabis Recommendations for Alzheimer's Disease

Recommending medical marijuana for patients with AD is a highly complicated matter. It can be challenging to convince other physicians and administrators that it's a good idea. While people with other chronic conditions can choose to use cannabis, most people with dementia don't have that option because the disease has robbed them of the ability to make educated medical decisions. Family members, caregivers, and other medical proxies may not have adequate information about—or interest in—making decisions about marijuana. And those patients living in nursing homes or other institutions are totally in the hands of the staff. Unfortunately, because of long-standing stigmas—and the dearth of clinical research—the use of marijuana for AD is especially slow to catch on. Even open-minded physicians and other healthcare workers may fear that medical marijuana will worsen their patients' memory, cause more symptoms, and make patient care ever more difficult. But from my experiences, the reverse is often true. For one thing, contrary to popular belief, small doses of cannabis can improve rather than impair memory. And it can also have a calming effect.

Hannah, a ninety-three-year-old great-grandmother, had advanced AD and was living in a group home. She was becoming increasingly agitated, had no appetite, and was losing a lot of weight. She was also up all night and slept all day, and would repeatedly scream in the middle of the night, making her care very difficult. The facility even threat-

ened to discharge her because other residents couldn't sleep. I started her on low doses of sublingual full-extract hemp oil with 12.5 mg of CBD twice a day plus 2 mg of THC brownies at night, and gradually increased the dosage to 5 mg. Within four weeks, her agitation improved dramatically, she was able to sleep through the night, and she gained weight. As a bonus, staff members were very happy to not have to deal with her nighttime screams, and her fellow residents were finally able to have a peaceful night's sleep.

There are no simple rules about using cannabis for the symptoms of AD. In general, however, as the disease progresses, more THC is usually needed to help with new or worsening symptoms. I find that the actual THC doses for managing the symptoms vary a lot from patient to patient. The ease of delivery is also important. Edibles, such as chocolates or brownies, often work well for patients with very advanced AD. They may have a hard time swallowing pills or following instructions to keep sublinguals under their tongue long enough for adequate absorption. For patients who are able to swallow capsules, though, adding cannabis capsules to their bedtime meds can be the best way to avoid changing their routine and introducing new foods or tastes.

Route of delivery is also a key factor in the willingness of administrators and staff to use medical cannabis. For example, because they're legal, hemp-based CBD oils, capsules, or edibles can often be administered at facilities as "supplements." But getting facility directors to allow the administration of medical marijuana is not so easy in states where it's still illegal. In our DC area, things have eased up, and more and more facilities allow patients to use cannabis as long as it is not an inhaled form. At the George Washington University Hospital where I practice, patients who are admitted to the hospital who have a recommendation for medical cannabis are allowed to continue to use it orally, sublingually, or rectally.

CANNABIS FOR DEMENTIA[44]

SYMPTOMS	DIAGNOSIS	DOSAGE
Agitation, anxiety, insomnia, depression, aggression	Dementia	THC:CBD mixes Doses ranging from 1–10 mg of THC and 30–100 mg of CBD/day at twice daily frequency
Appetite stimulation for weight loss	Advanced Dementia	Inhaled, sublingual, or oral, variable dosing, can probably start with just 1–2 mg of THC

Reversing Alzheimer's Disease

In addition to the promising benefits of cannabis for AD, there are some key lifestyle changes and other approaches that also look extremely promising. Of special note is Dr. Dale Bredesen's research article, "Reversal of Cognitive Decline," which was recently published in *The Journal of Alzheimer's Disease & Parkinsonism*.[45] In it, he describes his protocol, ReCODE®, that has led to the reversal of symptoms in hundreds of patients with Alzheimer's disease. ReCODE positions AD as a very complex and diverse group of biological processes with different causes and risk factors. These include insulin resistance/hyperglycemia, toxicity from heavy metals, hormonal/nutritional deficiencies, sleeping disorders, and other abnormalities. Dr. Bredesen's research demonstrates that these risk factors can be successfully addressed by targeting the root causes of cognitive decline for each patient, without using medications. Instead of pharmaceuticals, the ReCODE protocol includes diet adjustments, supplements, and other lifestyle modifications. Dr. Bredesen's journal article documents the cognitive and other improvements in one hundred people, some of whom were my patients, who followed the ReCODE protocol for AD or other serious cognitive problems.

My colleagues and I have since successfully treated many additional patients using the ReCODE protocol. One of our case studies, which demonstrated how detoxifying mercury was able to reverse Alzheimer's disease, was published in another medical journal in 2020.[46] I'm currently in the process of collecting more data and plan to publish our additional findings.

I'm also in the planning stages of a research project that involves adding medical cannabis to the ReCODE protocol to see if we can observe additional benefits. While this work is in its infancy and requires substantial funding, I've been slowly moving forward with identifying collaborators and collecting observational data. One of the hardest things with AD research is that the time required to assess the effects of any treatment intervention is usually measured in months and even years. But given the devastation that Alzheimer's disease wreaks on patients and families, it's definitely worth the effort.

HIGH HOPES FOR THE FUTURE

I truly believe that medical cannabis is one of the most exciting topics and positive developments in the field of neurodegenerative disorders, especially Alzheimer's disease. As additional evidence comes in, medical marijuana is likely to become more widely accepted and recommended for the treatment of AD to improve patients' quality of life and be recognized as an invaluable tool in palliative care.

Palliative care involves relieving debilitating symptoms and improving the quality of life for patients with serious chronic conditions as well as terminal, incurable diseases. It is especially important for treating patients in the final stages of their lives. In addition to relieving their symptoms, palliative measures can enhance their emotional well-being, and medical cannabis is one of the most important tools physicians have in our palliative toolbox.

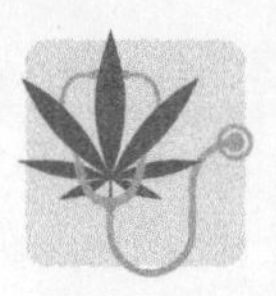

Hannah, the ninety-three-year-old grandmother mentioned above, who suffered from severe dementia, was rapidly deteriorating physically. Low-dose CBD and cannabis greatly improved her quality of sleep and decreased her anxiety and screaming outbursts. However, she became more paranoid and angry with the staff. Rather than prescribing the usual tranquilizers, in addition to her THC bedtime brownies, we gave her THC brownies in the morning and increased her daytime CBD. Beating all the odds, Hannah was able to celebrate her ninety-fifth birthday with her son before she passed away.

I strongly believe that the reason Hannah lived for two more years after we added medical cannabis to her treatment regimen was because her quality of life improved so much that she wanted to continue going on.

It's encouraging that medical cannabis is now becoming more acceptable for use in patients with life-threatening disease. As my colleague and cannabis expert Dr. Michelle Sexton and I wrote in our recently published journal article: "[M]ore and more patients suffering from incurable illnesses will turn to [medical cannabis] for relief of their symptoms. As clinical evidence grows, there is a good possibility that cannabis will one day become part of the standard palliative care toolbox."[47]

The need for medical cannabis in palliative medicine can't be underestimated. It's incumbent upon all of us healthcare professionals to do our best not only to make our patients comfortable, but also to help make their lives as pleasurable as possible. And medical marijuana has a major role to play in that pursuit.

CHAPTER TEN

Dealing with Doctors and Dispensaries

Even though medical marijuana is legal in most states, unless you live in a state with legalized recreational marijuana, obtaining it can be tricky business. If you live in a state that only has legal medical marijuana, you have to find a doctor or other healthcare provider who is certified to recommend medical marijuana. As we explained in Chapter 2, because marijuana is federally illegal, doctors can only *recommend* marijuana; they can't write a prescription for it. Once you get your recommendation, you then have to apply to your state health department to obtain a medical marijuana ID card, the magic key to getting medical marijuana.

DEALING WITH DOCTORS

Finding a Medical Marijuana Doctor

If you don't already have a recommendation, a good place to start is by asking your primary care physician (PCP) or other doctors if they are certified to recommend marijuana. If they aren't, ask them if they can refer you to someone who is. Explain why you believe that medical marijuana can you help with your condition, which, hopefully, is a qualifying condition in your state.

Qualifying Conditions

Qualifying conditions vary by state. It pays to know ahead of time what your state considers a qualifying condition by going to your state's health department or any of these websites:

- public.findlaw.com/cannabis-law/cannabis-laws-and-regulations/medical-marijuana-laws-by-state.html
- wayofleaf.com/mmj-cards/state/medical-marijuana-legal-states
- marijuanadoctors.com/medical-marijuana-doctors

As we mentioned in Chapter 2, chronic pain is by far the most common qualifying condition in all states.

Below are the most common qualifying conditions reported by patients (in alphabetical order):[1]

- Arthritis
- Cancer
- Chemo-induced nausea and vomiting
- Chronic pain
- Dementia
- Epilepsy
- Glaucoma
- HIV/AIDS
- Inflammatory bowel disease (IBD)

- Loss of weight and appetite
- Multiple sclerosis muscle spasms
- Post-traumatic stress disorder (PTSD)

But there are many other conditions that some states may consider as qualifying. For example, Illinois has one of the longest lists, with more than sixty. In addition to the ones mentioned above, they list migraines, Parkinson's disease, Tourette syndrome, autism, agitation of Alzheimer's disease, and opioid dependence, among many others.[2]

Bringing a list of your state's qualifying conditions can strengthen your argument. Such a list may also help educate your doctor about the benefits of medical marijuana. If your doctor is adamantly opposed to your using marijuana, find out why. Is it contraindicated for someone with your condition, or would it interact negatively with your other medications? If so, those are issues to take into serious consideration. But if your doctor is just opposed to pot in general, move on . . . and perhaps recommend this book to them!

If you're still looking for a doctor who can recommend cannabis, there are several good resources for finding certified cannabis specialists, including your state health department and cannabisclinicians.org

Consulting Costs

Not only can obtaining medical marijuana be a tricky business, it can also be a costly one. Even before you get to the point of buying it in a dispensary, there are considerable costs. First, there's the cost of consulting a medical marijuana doctor—or multiple doctors if you have trouble getting a recommendation. Insurance may not cover these appointments, which can run as high as $250 a visit or even more in some places. When you call for an appointment, ask about fees: Does the doctor charge by the visit or the hour? Do they take your insurance? Many states also require that patients' recommendations be renewed annually, which requires another doctor's visit . . . and another fee.

Meeting Your Marijuana Doctor

Once you've scored an appointment with a marijuana specialist, your visit should be just like going to any other doctor. It's a good idea to send your relevant medical records—including all your prescription and over-the-counter medications—ahead of time. If not, bring them with you; it will save a lot of time . . . and money. Any legitimate doctor will spend time with you to evaluate your medical situation to help determine whether medical marijuana is warranted. This is important because you want to make sure that you can safely use it. Depending on your presenting problem, some physicians may want to physically examine you to ascertain your state of health, as well as determine if you have a qualifying condition. This is yet another good reason to familiarize yourself with your state's qualifying conditions ahead of time.

Video Consultations

Because of the COVID-19 pandemic, more than half the states with legalized medical marijuana allowed doctors to evaluate patients who are seeking a recommendation for medical marijuana via video.[3] Patients and physicians alike have been happy about such virtual visits and hope that they outlast the pandemic. But some doctors and others fear that marijuana telemedicine has the potential for exploitation by patients who really just want to use pot for recreational purposes, as well as by physicians who want more patients for financial reasons.

In general, I strongly support the concept of video consults, but they're also not ideal in some situations, especially when a patient has a complex medical situation that might warrant a physical exam. However, when patients are referred by their doctors and their medical histories and diagnoses are clear, video consults with well-versed cannabis clinicians are actually a good way to go. For one thing, patients don't need to travel, which can be a financial and time concern for many. Video consults with cannabis doctors are also useful for follow-up questions and issues patients may have about medical marijuana. Most of what we do in medical cannabis is counseling, and 100 percent of this can be done on video. Patients can actually show the doctor all the cannabis products they're using and discuss content, dosing, and routes, etc. Of course, all of this depends on whether the physician has the necessary knowledge to discuss these issues. Lack of knowledge is a major issue that we cover later in this chapter.

Although some cannabis doctors offer videos consults to out-of-state patients, I strongly suggest that all patients consult a physician in their home state, for both legal and practical reasons. Video consults usually allow patients to get their medical marijuana ID card, which is much easier to do when using in-state physicians. They'll be familiar with your state laws and have access to the required forms. It's also easier for patients to get insurance reimbursement for in-state video consults, even if the doctor doesn't directly take their insurance. In any case, I believe that video consults are here to stay even after COVID and that most cannabis consults in the future will be conducted over video.

Dealing with Rejections

If a certified cannabis doctor refuses to write you a letter of recommendation, try to find out why. As mentioned above, marijuana is sometimes counterindicated for patients with certain medical conditions and/or when combined with certain other drugs. You can try to find another more cooperative doctor, but if that doctor agrees with the first one, medical marijuana may not be the best choice for your particular problem. To play it safe, it's best to discuss the issue with your other doctors, even though they may not be familiar with medical marijuana.

Dealing with Your Other Doctors

Whether or not you get a recommendation for marijuana, it's important to be open with your other physicians about your plans to use marijuana. It may help to bring a copy of this book with the sections relevant to your medical condition highlighted. According to a recent survey of primary care physicians and their patients, the PCPs were aware of marijuana use in only a little more than half of their patients who said they used marijuana.[4] Of their patients who they knew were using marijuana, the PCPs reported that almost a third of those patients had conditions for which they believed cannabis should be counterindicated.

The doctors you regularly see who are not marijuana specialists may give you the green light or raise legitimate concerns about the effect of cannabis on your medical condition or possible interactions with your other medications. If the latter is the case, or if you feel that your doctor just doesn't get it, you may want to get a second opinion. You might also suggest to these other doctors that they discuss the issue with your medical marijuana doctor. It may turn out to be an enlightening experience.

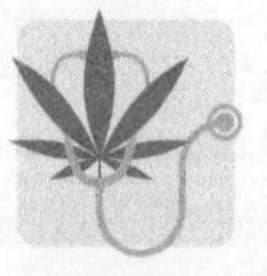

Dorothy, a seventy-six-year-old retired teacher, was admitted to our hospital because she had become delirious, a very serious side effect of gabapentin, a commonly used prescription drug she was taking for peripheral

neuropathy pain. I recommended that once she was weaned off gabapentin, she should try acupuncture and medical cannabis. Twelve weeks later, Dorothy was happy to report that both the acupuncture and pot helped relieve her pain. But then she added, "My primary care doctor wants you to call him. He thinks I should stop using pot as it is dangerous at my age. He wants me to take Lyrica medication instead . . . but I don't think so." She was wise to turn it down; Lyrica is similar to gabapentin but can have even more serious side effects in older adults. Plus, it's a controlled substance! I called her doctor to discuss her case and emailed him a journal article with a chart that graphically demonstrated how safe cannabis was compared to many commonly prescribed painkilling drugs. He was totally surprised by the data and has since been referring patients to me for management of chronic pain.

What to Expect from Your Medical Marijuana Doctor

Ideally, the doctor who agrees to give you a recommendation will also give you advice about what form of cannabis you should use, at what dosage, and by what route. But, realistically, most certifying cannabis physicians won't be able to give you this kind of specific advice. According to a number of surveys, the majority of these doctors, as well as PCPs, admit that they lack sufficient knowledge about marijuana to adequately counsel their patients about it.[5] One recent survey of medical marijuana doctors found that most got their information through conferences, journal articles, and/or websites, respectively.[6] But only a little more than half said that the information they received was sufficient to practice good cannabis medicine. So rather than giving you inadequate or incorrect information, your recommending doctor is likely to suggest that you get this important information from your dispensary. What your doctor can provide is an official letter or a certificate stating that you're qualified to use medical marijuana. This coveted document will enable you to get the all-important medical marijuana ID card.

MEDICAL MARIJUANA ID CARDS

Medical marijuana ID cards (MMICs) allow you to buy cannabis from a dispensary and, in some states, to grow your own pot. Each state has its own application process and application fees, which can vary from zero to as much as $200. It typically takes a week or longer to receive the card. In the DC/Maryland area where I practice, it takes on average more than four weeks to obtain an MMIC. This often causes significant problems for patients, especially when they're looking for quick symptom relief. Luckily, some of my patients in hospice care or with documented terminal illnesses have been able to get an expedited card in about twenty-four hours. Also, since the COVID pandemic, many states now allow online applications so patients can avoid standing in line. This can speed up the application process to about fifteen minutes. Most states require MMICs to be renewed each year for an additional charge. It may also involve another trip to your medical marijuana doctor or a video consultation—and another bill to pay.

MMICs are required in the states that have only legalized medical marijuana, but not in the states that have also legalized recreational pot. The numbers keep changing as more states in both categories are getting on the legalization bandwagon, so check your state's health department's website to see where your state stands. Regardless of whether you live in a legalized medical or recreational state, there are some important issues to consider if you are planning to use an MMIC.

Disadvantages of MMICs

Because marijuana is federally illegal, having a state-issued medical marijuana card may create some problems for you that can impact your career and civil rights:

- You cannot possess a commercial driver's license.
- You cannot hold a federal government job.
- You cannot possess a firearm.

Now for the pros, which outweigh the cons for most people:

Advantages of MMICs

- You are exempt from paying a marijuana sales tax (which can be as high as 37 percent!).
- You can buy products with much higher levels of THC and in larger quantities than recreational users.
- If you're under twenty-one, you can get medical marijuana with your parents' consent.
- You may pay less for medical marijuana and/or get special discounts.
- You can grow your own weed with few restrictions.
- You can use your card to buy pot in some other states.

Reciprocity

More and more states are granting reciprocity to out-of-state patients with MMICs to allow them to buy marijuana in their states. The laws vary, so check with the state you're visiting to see if it has reciprocity and what, if any, restrictions might apply. Americans for Safe Access (ASA) recommends that when you visit that state you keep a copy of your doctor's letter of recommendation and your MMIC with you at all times and keep another copy in your luggage.[7] ASA also suggests having copies of your physicians' and lawyers' numbers with you as well.

Last but not least, do not bring *any* form of cannabis with you when visiting the other (or any) state, and do not bring home any cannabis product you buy there. It's against the law!

Bad Trips

Traveling with marijuana across state lines can land you in jail! Even if you have an MMIC and marijuana is legal in the state you're traveling to, it's still illegal. While some cops may look the other way, it's not worth the risk. Crossing state lines with even small amounts of pot is a federal crime. The penalties for first offenders who transport less than 50 kg of pot—even one joint—can be up to five years in prison and $250,000 in fines![8] It's not fair, but it's the reality of the justice system as it is right now.

If you ignore or forget this advice and get pulled over by the police, Americans for Safe Access advises that you do not give them permission to search your car . . . unless they smell pot! If they do, they have probable cause to search your car. If they don't smell pot, and they persist in trying to search your car, state loudly and clearly, "I do not consent to a search." The good news is that if the search continues, it will be considered illegal and inadmissible in court.[9]

Traveling with marijuana to or from other countries, especially Canada, can also be risky. According to Canadian law, even if you are traveling from a US state that has legalized weed, crossing the border with any amount of cannabis is a criminal offense in deference to US federal laws.[10]

Flying with marijuana (but not flying high) appears to be safer than driving with pot in your possession; TSA agents are more interested in intercepting bombs and weapons than drugs.[11] But then again, if found, your marijuana can be confiscated, and you may face criminal charges. Check ahead of time with your airline and your destination country about their specific regulations.

Whether you're driving or flying, you have to weigh the risks and benefits for yourself and your medical situation. Only you can decide whether traveling with medical marijuana is worth the risk of arrest or having it confiscated. It may be wiser to wait to get your cannabis in a dispensary in a state (or country) where it's legal.

DEALING WITH DISPENSARIES

It's essential that all medical marijuana patients find dependable dispensaries that have the cannabis products they need, as well as a reliable sales staff (aka budtenders). Dispensaries are considered so indispensable that during the COVID pandemic, they were, like pharmacies, considered essential services.

That said, not all dispensaries are alike. Some are very aggressive about pushing their products. And the recommendations they make may be based on their recreational use rather than their medicinal value. Others may fail to store their products properly; marijuana is a plant and prone to mold, which can be toxic. And many cannabis products are not adequately tested or labeled, which we discuss later in this chapter.

Patients (and their doctors) also have to trust that the advice given by the budtenders is sensible and safe. But budtenders are salespeople, *not* healthcare professionals. Although most are undoubtedly sincere about helping clients, some may be just selling hype. Therefore, patients may need to take some of their advice with a grain of salt.

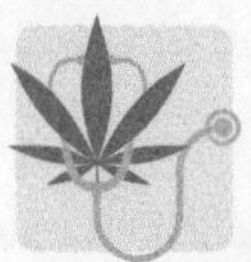

Sophia, the jewelry designer who had breast cancer (see Chapter 8), suffered from severe nausea from chemotherapy. She was lucky that her regular doctor was a cannabis-certified physician and was willing to write her a recommendation for medical marijuana. But, unfortunately, he couldn't provide her any guidance about what she should use. He told her that she should get the information from the dispensary. "I checked out about five different dispensaries but found them all weird." Her options were very confusing, with such colorful names as Chewy's Breath (high THC, low CBD), Vanilla Berry Pie (high THC, no CBD), Cherrygasm (low THC, high CBD), and countless other cannabis compounds. She didn't know if she should smoke or vape it, swallow it, put it under her tongue, rub it in, insert it, eat it, or drink it! When she told the budtenders that she had breast cancer, they were overly aggressive in promoting their products and exaggerating the benefits of pot. "They were all telling me to take a very strong THC oil that I read could be dangerous and can get you very high—like an LSD trip! I just wanted the nausea to go away!"

What to Expect from a Dispensary

What a dispensary is like often depends on the clientele as well as the state, city, and even the neighborhood it's in. In states that have only legalized medical marijuana, like New Mexico, the clientele is more likely to be older and have more chronic health problems than the customers in dispensaries in California, where recreational marijuana is legal. For example, a dispensary in a trendy city like Santa Fe, New Mexico, might resemble an upscale health food store or health spa, with comfortable chairs, healthy snacks, exotic flowers, and informational brochures. To get to the inner sanctum where the weed is kept, you have to present your medical marijuana card. The budtenders realize that the customers, at least most of them, are there to get relief from various symptoms, not to get high. Their ads, like the following, make it clear that they're targeting patients and not potheads: "Mother Nature called, your medicine is ready" and "Our mission is to help provide patients with the medicine they need; we are here because of you!"

On the other hand, dispensaries in California are quite different. For one thing, you don't need a medical marijuana card to buy weed. A dispensary in downtown San Francisco might look like a hippie head shop from the '60s . . . only with a guard outside. They do, after all, have age limits. But once inside, you'll see the pot products and paraphernalia openly displayed, waiting to be purchased by people who most likely want to get high . . . or very relaxed. Some dispensaries in other neighborhoods, however, might have a posh, sleek modern, or cozy clublike atmosphere that would appeal to a more upscale clientele. One dispensary describes itself as a "safe, clean, comfortable atmosphere for our clients to browse, get helpful recommendations, and relax and enjoy recreational cannabis." And some target clients who are clearly more interested in the medicinal benefits, as does this dispensary that offers its patrons "an unmatched curated selection of high-quality, award-winning, and lab tested cannabis brands and products . . . for health and wellness."

Check out dispensaries' websites carefully before visiting. You'll get a good sense of what their atmosphere, staff, and clientele are like. Then take a look inside and try to talk to a budtender or two.

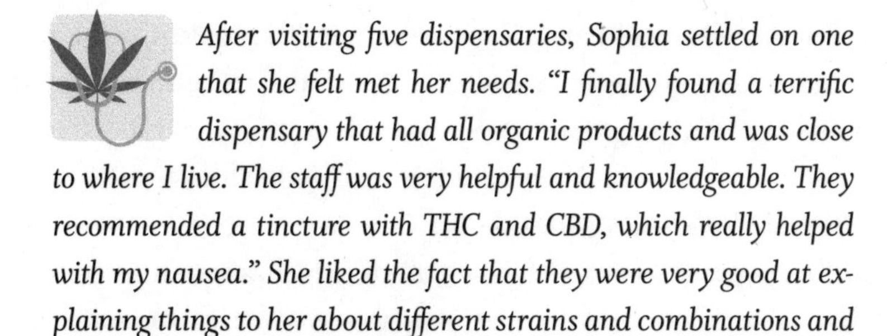

After visiting five dispensaries, Sophia settled on one that she felt met her needs. "I finally found a terrific dispensary that had all organic products and was close to where I live. The staff was very helpful and knowledgeable. They recommended a tincture with THC and CBD, which really helped with my nausea." She liked the fact that they were very good at explaining things to her about different strains and combinations and

that they had a lot of educational brochures about marijuana, which she found useful. She was especially grateful that they offered discounts to cancer patients because health insurance doesn't pay for medical marijuana. "They even give us a free joint for our birthdays," she said. And she liked the fact that they often donated part of their sales to local charities or events. Sophia also enjoys going to the dispensary. "It's like an elegant senior center with leather furniture and beautiful flowers," she explained. "They also have happy hours and holiday parties with free samples of marijuana-laced cookies, candies, and beverages!" Although Sophia said that some of the clients are "old hippies," most are well-dressed professionals, housewives, artists, and retirees in their sixties and seventies.

There are many other factors that you might want to consider when choosing a dispensary.

Location, Location

Convenience is a major consideration for many people. So having a dispensary close to home or work can be a big plus. Traveling many miles to get marijuana can be time-consuming and put a dent in your budget.

Home Delivery

States are increasingly allowing dispensaries to offer home delivery as well as curbside pickup services in yet another COVID cannabis concession. As with video consultations, these services are extremely popular and likely to remain after the pandemic is over. Check your state's health department website or ask your local dispensaries if home delivery is an option.

Dispensary-Grown Marijuana

Some dispensaries grow their own weed, which gives them control over their products' production, purity, and storage, among other advantages. And customers can learn a lot about the cannabis products before buying them. The budtenders are usually well informed about how the grass is grown, what pesticides—if any—are used, and the cannabinoid and terpene content of the products, among other key concerns. These "farm-to-table"—or more accurately, "farm-to-toke"—dispensaries are sometimes located on or near the dispensary and may have sampling and tasting rooms for clients. Many are also on the "cannabis tour circuit," which operates very much like vineyard tours. But the grass isn't always greener at dispensary gardens. While many of these farms are strictly organic and have their own testing labs, others may skimp on purity and quality to save money.[12] It pays to ask.

Pot Products

Dispensaries usually display a huge potpourri of pot products for you to choose from, and deciding what form of cannabis to use is a major challenge for most customers. The dispensary may have promotional brochures touting the benefits of their products, which may or may not be proven. Unfortunately, there are no national guidelines or regulations for cannabis products. The rules that do exist vary from state to state, so there are no standard dosages or quality control. As a result, patients have to trust that the products that dispensaries sell are safely stored and free from fungus, pesticides, and other toxins, as well as accurately labeled.

You're also likely to be inundated with ads and other information—often inaccurate—about medical marijuana through friends and social media. While often well meaning, much of the information on social media is pot propaganda or based on personal, anecdotal experiences rather than evidence. Some commercial cannabis sites also knowingly make exaggerated claims about their cannabis products. We hope that after reading this book, you'll have a better sense of what cannabis products you'd like to try *before* you go to the dispensary. That will send a message to the budtenders that you're an

MISLEADING MARIJUANA INFO

It's not just commercial sites that are the culprits in spreading marijuana misinformation. Even some government websites can't be trusted. In 2017, Americans for Safe Access (ASA)—a not-for-profit advocacy organization whose mission is to ensure safe and legal access to cannabis for therapeutic uses and research—forced the US Drug Enforcement Administration (DEA) to remove inaccurate, misleading information about the supposed harms of marijuana from their website and publications. The ASA had filed a legal complaint after it found more than twenty-five false statements on the DEA website alone.[13]

educated cannabis consumer, and that they should concentrate on your needs rather than on promoting their favorite products.

In states where medical marijuana is legal, you may also be able to get product information through the state's health department, or you can ask the dispensary for this information. Also, look at the label carefully to see if a product has been lab tested by a third-party independent lab. If it just says "lab tested," it might only be tested by the producer, and the results may not be objective or reliable.[14] If in doubt, you can request a copy of the third-party testing result from your dispensary. Hopefully, they will be able and willing to provide the information to you. Testing cannabis for contaminants and active ingredients has become routine and expected for all quality brands. Asking to verify that what you are consuming is safe and of good quality is your right as a consumer. It can also give you and your doctor much-needed peace of mind.

Deciphering Labels

You would think that labels are the most important part of the communication of what's in the dispensary product. And to a large degree, this is true. However, at present, there is no standard for labeling, and this is a huge problem. Requirements for labeling vary from state to state, so companies can choose what they want to put on the label. Key information, such as the presence of terpenes and minor cannabinoids like THCa and CBDa, may not be listed at all. Moreover, products sold online very often don't include exact ingredients; they may just show a photo of the bottle.

Arguably, the most information you will find on a label is the presence and amount of THC, CBD, other cannabinoids, and terpenes. But you should also look to see if there are additives such as certain oils, thinners, thickeners, color dyes, flavors, and other ingredients you wish to avoid. Unfortunately, this information is often missing. Ideally, cannabis products in all states should have labels that provide this information plus lot numbers, expiration dates, and other key information.

Reading product labels can help not only to ensure that you're getting a safe product, but also that you're getting the ingredients you need in the right ratios. However, reading and interpreting labels on cannabis products can be a quite a challenge. Consumers often complain about having difficulty interpreting labels and feeling overwhelmed by the all the information on them. To make matters worse, much of this information is printed on small bottles in a tiny font size.[15] And we all know how important reading the fine print can be!

Below are some sample labels and explanations of what they contain:

LABEL 1: CANNABIS VAPE CARTRIDGE

Lot: XXXXX-000000
Batch: CA20200612101
Expiration: June-11-2021

Black Afghan (500 mg)

Full Spectrum Cannabinoids:

THC	**75.7%**	**(378.5mg)**
CBG	**2.5%**	**(12.5mg)**
CBN	**1.0%**	**(5.0mg)**
CBC	**0.6%**	**(3.0mg)**

Strain-Specific Cannabis Terpenes: 5.15%

alpha-Pinene	0.29%
beta-Pinene	0.14%
beta-Myrcene	1.10%
D-Limonene	0.40%
Ocimene	0.22%
Terpinolene	0.07%
Fenchone	0.01%
Linalool	0.28%
Fenchol	0.10%
Borneol	0.13%
Terpineol	0.20%
Nerol	0.16%
beta-Caryophyllene	1.32%
alpha-Humulene	0.37%
Guaiol	0.08%
beta-Eudesmol	0.08%
alpha-Bisabolol	0.20%

ingredients: Medical Cannabis

Label 1 is on a box that contains a cannabis vape cartridge of full-spectrum cannabinoid, which includes most of the active ingredients in the cannabis plant. The main ingredient, THC 75.7 percent (378.5 mg), is listed first and the lesser cannabinoids are listed in descending order by percent and milligrams. Terpenes and other minor ingredients are listed in a very small font by percentage only. For information on the different cannabinoids and common terpenes, see Chapter 2.

LABEL 2: THC SUBLINGUAL TINCTURE

Lot: XXXXX-000000
Batch: CA20200528102
Expiration: May-27-2021

ENERGIZE TINCTURE

Cannabinoids:

THC	(100.8mg)
THCV	(3.8mg)
CBG	(2.0mg)

Cannabis Terpenes:

d-Limonene...... 0.20%

Label 2 is on the back of a small box of THC-predominant sublingual tincture. The front (not shown) just says Sativa Tincture THC 100 percent. The back label indicates that THC is the main ingredient. They only list one terpene, d-Limonene, because there's not enough space on the label to list all the ingredients, or because this is the only terpene in any measurable amount in the tincture.

LABEL 3: (FRONT) CBD OIL

CBD OIL

1000 MG • 1 OZ (30 ML)

The only information on the front of this tiny bottle, besides the manufacturer, is that it contains 1 ounce of 1000 mg of CBD oil. The rest of the information is on the back label shown below.

LABEL 3: (BACK) CBD OIL

Ingredients: Organic Extra Virgin Olive Oil, Full Spectrum Hemp Extract.

These statements have not been evaluated by the Food & Drug Administration. This product is not intended to diagnose, treat, cure, or prevent any disease.

The back of the bottle—if you can read the fine print—indicates that the main (inactive) ingredient is organic olive oil, which is mixed with the active ingredient, full-spectrum hemp extract (1000 mg as indicted on the front). In addition to containing CBD, full-spectrum hemp oil also contains trace amounts of THC and other cannabinoids, as well as terpenes, none of which are listed on the label, mostly due to lack of regulation and to minimize possible confusion. Lack of space is another problem. The fine print on the bottom states: "These statements have not been validated by the Food & Drug Administration. This product is not intended to diagnose, treat, cure, or prevent any disease." This type of warning is commonly found on supplements, including CBD derived from hemp and hemp products that are sold without restrictions. They are not federally illegal because they only contain trace amounts of THC—less than the 0.3 percent cutoff. CBD derived from cannabis, on the other hand, is federally illegal because it can contain more than 0.3 percent THC (see Chapter 2). It's also much more expensive than hemp-derived CBD.

LABEL 4: (FRONT) TOPICAL CBD SALVE

CBD SALVE
FULL SPECTRUM
300 MG CBD • NET WT. 2 OZ

The front of this label explains only that this topical contains 300 mg of full-spectrum CBD.

LABEL 4: (BACK) CBD TOPICAL SALVE

For topical use only.
Do not apply to broken skin.

Ingredients: Olive oil (infused with arnica, calendula, and chamomile*), shea butter*, beeswax, jojoba oil*, full-spectrum hemp extract*, lavender essential oil*, eucalyptus essential oil*, peppermint essential oil*, and vitamin E. *Organic

The back label describes the major ingredients in descending order from highest to lowest percentage. The CBD is described halfway down as full-spectrum hemp extract. It's important to carefully read the other ingredients to rule out any that you may be allergic to. Several of the ingredients listed, such as calendula, arnica, and eucalyptus, may be especially helpful for chronic pain and other health problems.

UNIVERSAL LABELING OF CANNABIS PRODUCTS

The solution to these labeling problems is to have universal labeling. I'm a founding physician member of Doctors for Cannabis Regulation (DFCR),[16] an organization that promotes cannabis legalization for adults, preventive education of minors, and regulation of the industry. Dr. David Nathan, the founder and board president, spearheaded a project to promote universal cannabis labeling. He recently issued a report in which he proposes the following two universal labels: a universal cannabis product symbol and a universal cannabis information label:[17]

PROPOSED UNIVERSAL CANNABIS PRODUCT SYMBOL

This symbol ideally would appear on the outside of all packages containing cannabis to caution adults and children that the product contains cannabis. The symbol would also be a guarantee that the product was legal and properly tested.

PROPOSED UNIVERSAL CANNABIS INFORMATION LABEL

Cannabis Information

Strain: **Sopheli OG** (Indica dom. Hybrid)
Product form: **Flower**
How it's used: **Inhaled**
Weight: **3.5g**
Serving size: **166mg***
Servings per container: **21**

*Serving size based on estimated inhalation and absorption of 10mg of heated Total THC. Serving size for flower consumed orally is 40% of the number shown. Actual ingestion may vary significantly.

← Strain name (required), Sativa v. Indica (optional), key product information

← QR link to online product and safety info

← Information on serving calculation

Cannabinoids Per Serving

Total THC	**15.1%**	**10.0mg**
THCA	2.3%	1.5mg
Total CBD	**13.4%**	**8.9mg**
CBDA	1.4%	0.9mg

Other cannabinoids (mg/serving):
CBN 0.63, CBG 0.30

Terpenes & flavonoids (mg/serving):
ß-Caryophyllene 3.4, Myrcene 2.5, Linalool 0.2, Limonene 7.7, a-Humulene 2.3, a-Pinene 1.9, ß-Pinene 1.0

← THC and CBD data per serving (required)

← Other cannabinoid, terpene, and flavonoid data per serving (optional)

← Ingredients or inactive ingredients (for concentrates, edibles, beverages, topicals, and suppositories)

WARNINGS: Keep out of reach of children and pets. This product may be addictive. Do not drive or operate machinery while intoxicated. This product may pose significant health risks to pregnant or breastfeeding women, minors, and people with psychiatric disorders.

← Health warnings (vary based on product form)

Lot **XXXXX-000000** Exp **04/18/23**

← Unique lot/tracking number and expiration date

Such universal symbols are especially important now that medical and/or recreational cannabis is legal in most states. As Dr. Nathan explained, "As the US federal government and individual states move toward full legalization of cannabis for adults, the regulation of cannabis product labeling is essential to ensure the protection of public health and safety."[18]

Universal labeling is also the best way consumers can guarantee that they're getting what they paid for.

MONEY MATTERS

Doses and Dollars

It's not only important to understand how much THC, CBD, and other cannabinoids are in each dose but also how many doses are in each bottle and how much each dose actually costs. That way you can comparison shop and get the best bang for your buck!

Determining such information can be quite challenging and time-consuming, but the good news is that a nonprofit organization devoted to cannabis for autism, Whole Plant Access for Autism, has an easy-to-use calculator to help you figure it out: wpa4a.org/wpa4a-calculators/price-per-mg-calculator/.

Insurance

Costs are a major consideration for most people who use medical marijuana. Unfortunately, health insurance—including Medicare and Medicaid—doesn't cover the cost of medical marijuana. This is yet another negative consequence of cannabis's designation as a Schedule I federally illegal substance. Understandably, insurance companies can't reimburse the costs of illegal drugs. Additionally, insurance companies can only cover drugs for which doctors write prescriptions. And doctors are forbidden to write cannabis prescriptions; they can only recommend it. Another catch-22!

Americans for Safe Access (ASA) and other advocacy groups are fighting hard to get cannabis rescheduled as a medicine so that, among other advantages, it can be covered by insurance.[19] ASA conducted a large survey and found that affordability is the most serious challenge medical marijuana users face.[20] In fact, almost 90 percent of those surveyed said that the cannabis they needed was not affordable.[21]

Another major roadblock to the efforts to have marijuana covered by insurance is that only drugs that are listed in the National Formulary can be covered . . . and these drugs have to have FDA approval. That's why insurance companies can reimburse FDA-approved synthetic and other cannabis-derived pharmaceutical drugs, such as Marinol and Cesamet (see Chapter 2).[22] Ironically, their costs are sky-high compared to naturally grown weed sold in dispensaries, which patients prefer by far.

Realistically, the only way the FDA would approve natural cannabis products sold in dispensaries is if they were produced by Big Pharma, and that would take many years of clinical trials and millions of dollars. And those costs would, of course, be passed on to the consumer.[23] For example, the average cost of Marinol for a year can be more than $8,000, depending on insurance coverage.[24] So even if insurance ultimately paid for some of the costs, the copays would undoubtedly be higher than the cost of dispensary marijuana.

Cash Only

Be prepared to pay cash when you buy cannabis. This is yet another annoying consequence of marijuana being federally illegal. Banks and credit card companies are understandably not keen on getting involved in illegal money activities! While a few dispensaries may have arrangements with local banks, the majority require cash. If you're lucky, there will be an ATM on, site or nearby. But that may involve paying a service fee.

Cost-Saving Strategies

The cost of cannabis products is all over the place; it depends on what state you live in and even where in that state you buy your marijuana. You might want to check out priceofweed.com which provides nationwide and statewide price information for marijuana. Another website, weedmaps.com/learn/cbd/how-much-does-cbd-oil-cost-what-you-need-to-know, has useful information on the price of CBD.

Dispensaries can charge what they want, so you'll have to do your own comparison shopping in your community if you want to get the best deal. The easiest way is to look online or call several different dispensaries and ask about the costs of your preferred products.

Discounts: Dispensaries often give discounts for client referrals and to seniors, cancer patients, veterans, and loyal customers.

Coupons: Many cannabis websites have coupons you use online in states where buying online is allowed.[25] Check with your dispensary to see if they'll accept your coupons.

Grow your own: If you're a DIY person—or just into gardening—this may be a good way to save money. Just be sure to check with your state about their regulations, especially how much you can grow for personal use.

Some people also advocate buying in bulk to save money. But it's best to avoid purchasing large amounts of a specific cannabis product since most patients need to try several different ones before identifying what works best. What's more, you may end up using two to four different products depending on your specific needs, which may change over time.

DEALING WITH BUDTENDERS: YOUR NEW BESTIES

Once you've settled on a dispensary (or two), it's important to find budtenders you trust to help you navigate the complicated world of medical cannabis. They can help you decide what products to use, in what dose, and by what route. This is especially important because, as we mentioned above, most doctors, including those who are certified to recommend cannabis, tend to have limited knowledge on the subject.

While budtenders play an extremely critical role in advising patients about medical marijuana, they are, as we have said, salespeople, not healthcare professionals. While physicians, nurses, pharmacists, and other health-care providers go through specialized training before giving out medical advice, budtenders aren't required to take any cannabis-related courses, much less have any medical training. In one national survey, only 20 percent of budtenders had taken any medically oriented courses or training in cannabis.[26] However, many budtenders—especially those who work in medical dispensaries—do get some sort of training. A survey of budtenders in Oregon found that almost all of the respondents said they learned about medical marijuana through on-the-job training. Almost one in three also attended cannabis-related conferences, and the internet was a major source of information for many.[27] While most budtenders had some college education, very few had an academic background in health or other sciences.

In spite of not having a medical background, the reality is that many budtenders know much more than the average MD about medical marijuana. So, by default, budtenders are filling a critical role in patient education that normally would be the responsibility of doctors. Dr. Donald Abrams, an oncologist and renowned expert on cannabis (see Chapter 8), recommends medical marijuana to many of his patients. However, even he sometimes relies on budtenders to give his patients advice on the specific strains to use. As he explained, "They're on the front lines."[28]

Doctor-Budtender Communication

Unfortunately, there's often a disconnect between recommending physicians and budtenders, which can be problematic for patients. According to a recent journal article: "Inadequate and inconsistent communication between certifying physicians and dispensary staff leads to conflicting advice on MC [medical cannabis] strength of dose, frequency of use, route of administration, cannabinoid and terpene profile, and strain selection."[29]

Getting the right balance and dosage of THC and CBD is especially critical for older adults and those who have cancer or other serious diseases. For example, too high a dose could cause blood pressure to fall dangerously low or rise too high. And the wrong strain could make a person too drowsy—increasing the risks of falls—or too hyper—increasing anxiety or panic attacks. When doctors and budtenders are on the same page, it can help ensure that patients get the appropriate product and dose, as well as avoid potentially serious side effects and negative interactions with other medications.

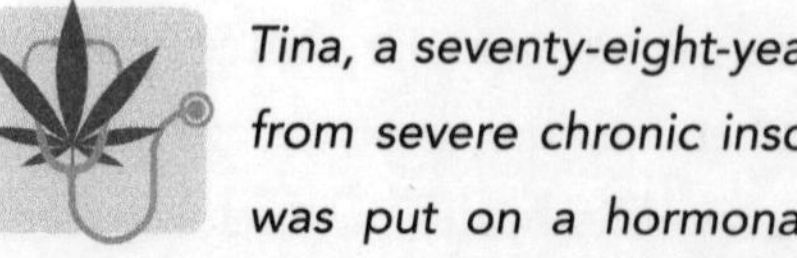

Tina, a seventy-eight-year-old retired nurse, suffered from severe chronic insomnia that started after she was put on a hormonal medication that prevents breast cancer recurrence. I recommended that she try a low-dose

sublingual THC tincture, which she got at her local dispensary. But the first night she took it, her insomnia worsened. She had developed a paradoxical reaction—a bad reaction to the combination of the two drugs. Unaware of this, the dispensary told her to double her dose of the THC tincture. That night she didn't sleep at all. The following morning, she felt beyond miserable and fell down and fractured her wrist. When she finally contacted me, I explained that she had had a bad reaction to the combination of drugs and told her to stop all THC-containing products. I recommended a low-dose, full-spectrum, hemp-derived CBD, which helped her sleep better. While the recommendation made by the dispensary clerk to double the dose may have made some sense for someone twenty years younger, a nonmedical provider is highly unlikely to recognize such a paradoxical reaction in an older patient.

Tina's story demonstrates that no matter how experienced a budtender is, patients shouldn't totally rely on them for more complex medical situations. Unfortunately, their recommending physicians may know even less. It's a Catch 22 situation. Another problem is that many patients have a hard time communicating some pertinent information to budtenders about their medical condition. Like Tina, they might just say they're having trouble sleeping, when the situation is more complicated. And the budtender might not ask some relevant questions, such as what other meds the person is taking or whether pain is also part of the picture.

Tina's story also highlights the importance of budtenders and physicians collaborating, especially when older, sicker patients are involved.

On-Site Medical Staff

The future of medical cannabis treatment will be based on effective teamwork. I'm a strong believer that *every* dispensary should have a medical provider on board. It could be a pharmacist, nurse, physician's assistant, or any other healthcare worker. But it has to be somebody with knowledge about and clinical experience with medical cannabis.

Although there's a trend toward having more doctors or other healthcare professionals on staff at dispensaries, it's not mandatory in most states. A few states do have very specific requirements, though. Maryland, for example, requires that all dispensaries have a medical clinical director, who can be a physician, nurse, or virtually any health-care provider trained in the use of medical cannabis.[30] The clinical director is expected to provide quality education to patients, their caregivers, and the dispensary staff; must be on-site or available remotely; and is required to take a training course each year. In Arizona, dispensaries must have a physician as a medical director, and Connecticut requires that dispensaries have a licensed pharmacist as their facility manager.[31] Pennsylvania requires that an MD or pharmacist be on-site during dispensary business hours.[32] Unfortunately, these states are in the minority. In an ideal world, *all* dispensaries would have physicians, pharmacists, nurses, and mental health professionals who have knowledge and experience with medical marijuana available on-site or on call.

PHYSICIAN EDUCATION

To fill the major and unfortunate gap in knowledge about medical marijuana among physicians, mandatory continuing medical education (CME) or other evidence-based cannabis courses are urgently needed. As the author of a recent physician survey explained:[33]

> *All states that allow medical cannabis require a physician's recommendation, yet few states require specific clinical training. Findings of this study suggest the need for more formal education and training of physicians in medical school and residency, more op-*

portunities for cannabis-related continuing medical education for practicing physicians, and clinical and basic science research that will inform best practices in cannabis medicine.

In 2015, several of my colleagues and I collaborated in developing the first cannabis CME course for the Washington, DC, Department of Health. The good news is that since then an increasing number of certified cannabis specialists and other doctors who want to learn more about medical marijuana are choosing to take cannabis courses, which have now sprung up across the nation.

But as of publication, only a handful of states require that recommending physicians take a CME or some other course in medical cannabis. To see if cannabis CME courses are required or recommended in your state, check fsmb.org/siteassets/advocacy/key-issues/medical-marijuana-cme-requirements.pdf.

Lack of healthcare providers' education is such a big deal that in partnership with one of the top integrative medicine journals, *Complementary Therapies in Medicine*, I am working with Leslie Mendoza Temple from the University of Chicago and Richard Isralowitz and Yuval Zolotov from Ben-Gurion University in Israel on a special journal issue on the subject.[34] We want to not only provide the best available evidence about medical cannabis but also advocate for comprehensive education on the subject for healthcare professionals. We hope that our work and the work of others will lead to the formation of a standardized curriculum in all medical schools and allied healthcare fields. Physicians aren't the only ones who should be taking these evidence-based courses. Other healthcare professionals—including pharmacists, mental health workers, and medical and nursing students—need to get on the education bandwagon to help meet the needs of growing numbers of medical marijuana patients. And, last but not least, budtenders and other dispensary staff who interact with patients should be taking these courses as well.[35] As Dr. Abrams said, they're the ones on the front lines.[36]

All these proposed measures are not just pipe dreams; they're important, attainable improvements that are necessary to ensure that medical marijuana patients get evidence-based advice and safe, effective treatment. Cannabis education for patients is also essential. That's why we wrote this book.

As you've seen, medical cannabis can be a very complex and controversial subject. But it's also an immensely exciting one. Most states have legalized the use of medical marijuana, and even recreational use is becoming more acceptable . . . and legal. It's likely that in the near future, the designation of marijuana as a Schedule I illegal drug will be history. That means there will be even more large-scale clinical research studies that will validate the many health benefits of cannabis we discuss in this book and discover new ones as well.

Marijuana has had a long, arduous journey from starting out as a common cure to being reviled as the devil's weed to rapidly gaining acceptance in mainstream medicine. We hope that this book has helped you navigate the complicated medical, legal, and consumer world of medical cannabis. And we especially hope that your journey to find relief is a successful one.

APPENDIX I

Glossary of Terms

Anandamide: The first endocannabinoid (see below) that was discovered. It has the same structure and psychoactive effects as THC. Its name, anandamide, is a play on the Sanskrit word for supreme joy or bliss.

β-caryophyllene (BCP): A terpene (see below) commonly found in cannabis that has antioxidant, analgesic, and anti-inflammatory effects.

Bioavailability: The amount (percent) of a drug that enters your bloodstream and can reach its target site. The higher the percent, the better. Bioavailability depends on many factors, especially the route of delivery.

Broad-spectrum extracts (aka broad-spectrum CBD oil): Similar to whole-plant CBD oil, except that *all* the THC has been removed.

Cannabichromene (see CBC)

Cannabidiol (see CBD)

Cannabigerol (see CBG)

Cannabinoid receptors (see CB1 and CB2 receptors below)

Cannabinoids: Active chemicals found in cannabis. There are three types of cannabinoids: phytocannabinoids, endocannabinoids, and synthetic cannabinoids, which are described below.

Cannabinol (see CBN)

Cannabis: A substance derived from the cannabis plant that has more than 0.3 percent THC.

Cannabis plant: A plant that is a member of the *Cannabaceae* family, a small family of flowering plants that includes about 170 species.

Cannabis indica: A subspecies of cannabis that also contains more than 0.3 percent of THC, but in lesser amounts than *sativa*. However, it has higher levels of CBD and tends to have a calming effect, so it's best used in the evenings.

Cannabis ruderalis: A subspecies of cannabis that contains less than 0.3 percent THC but high levels of CBD.

Cannabis sativa: A subspecies of cannabis that contains more than 0.3 percent THC; it tends to have a stimulating effect and is best used during the day.

Cannabis sativa L: The scientific name of the cannabis plant.

CB1 receptors: Cannabinoid receptors that are found predominantly in the brain and spinal cord. They're responsible for pain control, coordination, cognition, emotions, and other central nervous system functions. THC activates CB1 receptors.

CB2 receptors: Cannabinoid receptors that are located in almost all body systems, especially the immune system, where they control inflammation. THC activates CB2 receptors.

CBC (cannabichromene): A nonintoxicating cannabinoid that has anti-inflammatory and analgesic effects. It also has sedative, anti-anxiety, and antidepressant benefits, and may counter the intoxicating effects of THC. In addition, it appears to have antifungal and antibacterial properties.

CBD (cannabidiol): One of the major cannabinoids derived from the cannabis plant. CBD has very low levels of THC (under 0.3 percent) and is therefore not intoxicating.

CBDa (cannabidiolic acid): The botanical precursor of CBD. CBDa is found in raw cannabis plants and only becomes CBD when heated. CBDa has been shown to be useful in treating nausea and anxiety and is also a potent anti-inflammatory and analgesic.

CBG (cannabigerol): A nonintoxicating cannabinoid that has been shown to reduce pain and inflammation. It also holds promise as an appetite stimulant and a treatment for some gastrointestinal problems, mood disorders, and neurological conditions. Even more impressive is that, according to some animal studies, it's able to inhibit the growth of certain cancers.

CBN (cannabinol): A close cousin to CBD, CBN has anti-inflammatory, analgesic, and anticonvulsive effects. It also has mild psychoactive effects and can act as a sedative, especially when used with THC.

Cesamet (see nabilone)

Delta-8: A form of THC (Delta-9) that is less psychoactive. Because it's typically derived from CBD, which is federally legal, it's widely sold as a legal drug. However, for now, it's designated as a Schedule I illegal drug, which is currently under review by the Drug Enforcement Agency (DEA).

Delta-9 tetrahydrocannabinol: The chemical name for THC.

Dronabinol (Marinol): A synthetic pharmaceutical-form THC that is FDA approved for chemotherapy-related nausea and vomiting, and as an appetite stimulant for AIDS and cancer patients. It is only available by prescription.

Endocannabinoids: Natural cannabis-like chemicals that are produced inside the human body. They can have the same physiological and psychoactive effects as cannabis when they activate certain receptors in the endocannabinoid system.

Endocannabinoid system (ECS): A major body system that is responsible for maintaining our health and metabolism. It affects every organ and cell in our bodies from our brains to our reproductive systems and plays a key role in regulating our metabolism, hormones, digestion, emotions, and nervous system, among others.

Entourage effect: A phenomenon in which the different components of the whole cannabis plant—especially THC, CBD, and terpenes—work together synergistically to produce increased therapeutic benefits.

Epidiolex (cannabidiol): Cannabis-derived CBD that is FDA approved for the treatment of rare and severe forms of epilepsy and other seizure disorders in children and adults. It is the only naturally derived cannabinoid with FDA approval and only available by prescription.

FECO oil (full-extract cannabis oil): FECO is whole-plant extract in oil form. It provides a very high potency cannabis that can be used by any route of delivery except for smoking.

First-pass effect (aka first-pass metabolism): A phenomenon that only affects the oral route of delivery—that is, pills and edibles. When cannabis (or any other drug) is ingested orally, it must "first pass" through the gastrointestinal system and liver, where it's metabolized (broken down) before reaching the bloodstream and the target tissue or organ. It's one of the most important factors in determining the bioavailability of oral THC and CBD and how quickly the effects are felt.

Flavonoids: Natural compounds found in cannabis and other plants that, like terpenes (see below) are responsible for a plant's fragrance and flavor. They also frequently contribute to a plant's color. Most flavonoids have antioxidant and anti-inflammatory properties.

Flower: The hairy or sticky parts of the female cannabis plant. Cannabis flower is the most popular form of marijuana, is high in THC, and is usually smoked or vaped.

Full-extract cannabis oil (aka FECO oil): See above.

Full-plant extracts: These extracts are very similar to full-spectrum extracts/whole-plant extracts (see below). However, full-plant extracts may contain additional natural ingredients such as vitamins, fibers, and other nutrients because it undergoes less processing than full-spectrum extracts.

Full-spectrum extracts (aka whole-plant extracts): These extracts have had the impurities removed from the cannabis plant, while maintaining all the active ingredients of the whole plant, including THC, CBD, other cannabinoids, and terpenes, among others.

Hashish: The highly concentrated and intoxicating resin derived from the cannabis plant.

Hemp (aka industrial hemp): A strain of the *Cannabis sativa* that is cultivated for seeds and fiber. Because hemp has only trace amounts of THC (under 0.3 percent), it's federally legal.

Hybrids: Hybrids are a combination of different strains of cannabis. Because of hybridization, there are now countless varieties of cannabis available, each with a different level of potency and effects.

Isolates: The purest form of THC, CBD, or other cannabinoids that is chemically extracted from the cannabis plant.

Limonene: A terpene (see below) that has anti-inflammatory, anticancer, and sedative effects.

Linalool: A terpene (see below) commonly found in cannabis that has sedative, anti-inflammatory, and analgesic effects.

Marijuana (aka marihuana): The most commonly used term for cannabis in the United States. Because marijuana contains more than 0.3 percent THC, it is psychoactive and federally illegal. (See THC.)

Marinol (see dronabinol)

Myrcene: A terpene (see below) commonly found in cannabis that has analgesic, anti-inflammatory, and sedative effects.

Nabilone (Cesamet): A synthetic pharmaceutical-form THC that is FDA approved for chemotherapy-related nausea and vomiting, and as an appetite stimulant for AIDS and cancer patients. It is only available by prescription.

Phytocannabinoids: Naturally derived chemicals from the cannabis plant. Of the more than 100 phytocannabinoids that have been identified, THC and CBD are the most well known and medically important ones.

Pinene: A terpene (see below) commonly found in cannabis that has anti-inflammatory, antibacterial, antiseptic, gastroprotective, and anticancer effects.

Rick Simpson Oil (RSO): A full-spectrum cannabis oil that is much higher in THC and/or CBD than most other full-spectrum oils.

Sativex (nabiximols): A pharmaceutical drug that contains natural THC and CBD. It helps control neuropathic pain and some of the symptoms of multiple sclerosis. Although approved for use in Europe and many other countries, as of publication, Sativex has not been approved by the FDA, so it is not available in the United States.

Schedule I drugs: A designation by the FDA that indicates that a drug has no currently accepted medical use and has a high potential for abuse and is therefore federally illegal. Marijuana or any form of cannabis with more than 0.3 percent THC is labeled a Schedule I drug. Other drugs in this category include heroin, LSD, and other hallucinogens.

Synthetic cannabinoids: Pharmaceutically developed drugs that mimic the effects of natural cannabinoids that are FDA approved and are only available by prescription. They include dronabinol (Marinol) and nabilone (Cesamet), which are described above.

Terpenes: A large group of oils found in cannabis and other plants that are responsible for a plant's distinctive aromas, flavors, and therapeutic effects. The five most common and popular terpenes in cannabis are β-caryophyllene, limonene, linalool, myrcene, and pinene.

Terpenoids: A term often used interchangeably with terpenes because they are very similar. However, one major distinction is that terpenes are wet while terpenoids have been dried out.

THC (Delta-9 tetrahydrocannabinol): The psychoactive ingredient in cannabis, commonly referred to as marijuana. In addition to its intoxicating effects, THC has anti-inflammatory, anti-anxiety, and analgesic effects. THC is federally illegal because it is still a Schedule I drug (see above). It can only be bought in states that have legalized medical or recreational marijuana.

THCa (tetrahydrocannabinolic acid): A nonpsychoactive cannabinoid found in the raw cannabis plant. It's actually the precursor to THC, and only converts to THC when activated by heat or light. It has anti-inflammatory, neuroprotective, anti-seizure, anti-nausea, and analgesic properties and is legal in most states.

THCV (tetrahydrocannabivarin): A relative of THC that's considered a minor cannabinoid because it's found only in trace amounts in some cannabis strains. At low doses it's not intoxicating, but at high doses it may enhance the psychoactive effects of THC. It also appears to boost the anti-inflammatory, anticancer, and analgesic effects of THC and other cannabinoids. THCV is not federally illegal.

Trichomes: Microscopic, mushroom-shaped, hairlike growths that protrude from the buds and flowers of the female cannabis plants. They produce high concentrations of cannabinoids, including THC and CBD, as well as terpenes (see above).

Vaping: A method of inhaling cannabis as a vapor rather than smoke. Cannabis flower or concentrate is heated in a vaporizing device (vaporizer) to a temperature below the point of combustion to produce a vapor.

Whole-plant extracts (aka full-spectrum extracts): See above.

APPENDIX II

Cannabis Resources

EDUCATIONAL AND ADVOCACY NONPROFIT WEBSITES

Americans for Safe Access

safeaccessnow.org

ASA provides training and resources for activists. Their site includes legal resources for each state and information on talking to the media, testifying, lobbying, movement building, and more. They also offer condition-based booklets and state legal manuals.

Cannabis Reports

cannabisreports.org

Cannabis Reports provides news and reviews on topics, including cannabis products, dispensaries, doctors, and lawyers, as well as articles on growing marijuana and cooking with cannabis.

Marijuana Policy Project

mpp.org

MPP's mission is to increase support for nonpunitive cannabis policies and support those working for these changes, including changes to state laws to eliminate penalties for cannabis and gain influence in Congress.

NORML

norml.org

NORML provides information about the personal, medical, and industrial use of cannabis. They also report on testing, health endorsements, legal issues, and research. State NORML chapters provide varying levels of education, primarily regarding legal issues.

Patients Out of Time (POT)

patientsoutoftime.com

POT provides information on cannabis to healthcare professionals, patients, and caregivers. They highlight clinical conferences, information about the therapeutic basis of cannabis, and indications for its use.

ProCon.org

procon.org

Procon is a nonprofit public organization that provides resources for critical thinking to educate without bias. Cannabis is one of many issues discussed on their website.

Project CBD

projectcbd.org

Project CBD is a nonprofit educational service dedicated to promoting research into the medical utility of cannabidiol (CBD) and other components of the cannabis plant. It is intended to update providers and patients about developments in cannabinoid science, publicize research, and emphasize whole-plant cannabis therapeutics (not just THC or CBD).

Veterans for Medical Cannabis Access

veteransformedicalmarijuana.org

VMCA is an educational and patient advocacy resource on medical cannabis–related veterans' issues, including chronic pain and PTSD. VMCA is committed to protecting the rights of veteran patients and healthcare professionals by advocating for safe and legal access to cannabis for all appropriate therapeutic uses and to encourage research on cannabis as a treatment alternative.

CANNABIS MEDICAL AND RESEARCH ORGANIZATIONS

AMERICAN ACADEMY OF CANNABINOID MEDICINE
aacm.info

AMERICAN CANNABIS NURSES ASSOCIATION
cannabisnurses.org

AMERICAN MEDICAL MARIJUANA PHYSICIANS ASSOCIATION
ammpa.net

DOCTORS FOR CANNABIS REGULATION
dfcr.org

INTERNATIONAL ASSOCIATION FOR CANNABINOID MEDICINES
cannabis-med.org

INTERNATIONAL CANNABINOID RESEARCH SOCIETY
icrs.com

SOCIETY OF CANNABIS CLINICIANS
cannabisclinicians.org

COMMERCIAL CANNABIS INFORMATION WEBSITES

We recommend the following commercial websites because they offer useful information about cannabis, but we do not endorse any of their products.

healer.com/cannabiseducation

leafly.com/news/cannabis-101

weed.com/articles/cannabis-101

DIY CANNABIS TOPICALS AND SUPPOSITORIES INFORMATION

leafly.com/news/strains-products/how-to-make-diy-cannabis-topicals

projectcbd.org/wellness/how-make-cbd-home-remedy-kit-and-why-you-should

projectcbd.org/medicine/do-cannabis-suppositories-work

FURTHER READING

Backes, Michael. *Cannabis Pharmacy: The Practical Guide to Medical Marijuana.* New York: Black Dog & Leventhal, 2017.

Danko, Danny. *A Beginner's Guide to Growing Marijuana.* Charlottesville, VA: Hampton Roads Publishing, 2018.

Green, Greg, *The Cannabis Grow Bible*, 6th ed. San Francisco: Green Candy Press, 2017.

Readers Digest and Project CBD. *The Essential Guide to CBD.* New York: Trusted Media Brands, 2021.

Werner, Clint. *Marijuana Gateway to Health: How Cannabis Protects Us from Cancer and Alzheimer's Disease.* San Francisco: Dachstar Press, 2011.

Wolfe, Laura. *The Cannabis Apothecary.* New York: Black Dog & Leventhal, 2020.

Acknowledgments

First and foremost, we would like to thank Susan Orlins, our marvelous matchmaker. Misha, an integrative geriatrician, was looking for a medical writer for a book on healthy aging for seniors, and Joan, a medical writer, was looking for a new project. Thanks to Susan, we were the perfect match for the book—a young geriatrician and an older medical writer/sociologist! Given the increasing interest in medical marijuana, especially among seniors, and the increasing evidence that it worked, we decided instead to write a book on that subject. Our wonderful agent, Kris Dahl, loved the idea! Thanks to Kris's suggestions and guidance, we found the perfect publisher, Avery, and terrific editors, Lucia Watson and Suzy Swartz. We can't thank them enough for their enthusiasm, suggestions, and patience. Many thanks to Sharon Gonzalez, who did a great job of copyediting, and the designers who helped produce a beautiful book. We also want to thank Nenad Jakesevic for his wonderful terpene drawings and Sonja Lamut for Joan's author photo.

A special thanks to Dr. Andrew Weil, Dr. David Nathan, and Dr. Donald Abrams for their personal encouragement and contributions to the book. We also thank Stephanie Kahn for sharing her father's poignant story with us. We wish we could personally acknowledge all the patients whose stories so enrich our chapters, but their identities need to be kept confidential.

Misha would personally like to thank Leslie Mendoza Temple, Richard Isralowitz, and Yuval Zolotov for spending countless hours thinking about and discussing how to improve education of our future doctors and other healthcare providers in regard to medical cannabis. Misha wants to specially thank Elizabeth Hayes for her contributions to the book and the many hours of her time she spent teaching him important aspects of helping patients learn how to best use medical cannabis. Lastly, Misha wants to thank George Washington University Office of Integrative Medicine and Health and the Center for Integrative Medicine, including Janette Rodriguez, Dr. Leigh Frame, Dr. Marianna Ledenac, Dr. Deirdre Orceyre, and his wife, Angela Gabriel, for helping with many medical cannabis–related research and educational projects. Misha also wants to thank Angela for protecting his time to work on the book and being a pillar of our family unit during the treacherous time of COVID-19.

Joan is especially grateful to her husband, Richard—an incredibly talented writer and editor—for his spot-on edits, insightful comments, and helpful suggestions, not to mention his creative cooking. His delicious dinners and perfect wine selections were immensely appreciated and necessary during the seemingly endless writing process and pandemic. Joan also wants to thank their daughter, Rebecca, who has inherited her father's editing skills: her input and insights were extremely helpful. More important, her skills as a psychiatric social worker were most impressive; she provided (mostly socially distanced) much-needed emotional and loving support during this past year.

Notes

FOREWORD

1. A. T. Weil, N. E. Zinberg, and J. M. Nelsen, "Clinical and Psychological Effects of Marijuana in Man," *Science* 162 (1968): 13; A. T. Weil and N. E. Zinberg, "Acute Effects of Marihuana on Speech," *Nature* 222 (1968): 434–437.
2. Mikhail Kogan, ed., *Integrative Geriatric Medicine* (New York: Oxford University Press, 2017).
3. https://integrativemedicine.arizona.edu/oxford_press.html.

INTRODUCTION

1. Integrative medicine treats the whole person, not just the disease. It emphasizes a healthy lifestyle and safe, non-pharmacological, evidence-based complementary and conventional treatments.
2. Seegehalli M. Anil et al., "Cannabis Compounds Exhibit Anti-inflammatory Activity In Vitro in COVID-19–related Inflammation in Lung Epithelial Cells and Pro-inflammatory Activity in Macrophages," *Scientific Reports* 11, no. 1 (2021): 1–14; Vinit Raj et al., "Assessment of Antiviral Potencies of Cannabinoids against SARS-CoV-2 Using Computational and In Vitro Approaches," *International Journal of Biological Macromolecules* 168 (2021): 474–485.

CHAPTER 1: THE LONG AND WINDING ROAD

1. Ernest L. Abel, *Marihuana: The First Twelve Thousand Years* (Berlin: Springer Science+Business Media, 1980; reprinted 2013).

2. Simona Pisanti and Maurizio Bifulco, "Medical Cannabis: A Plurimillennial History of an Evergreen," *Journal of Cellular Physiology* 234, no. 6 (2019): 8342.
3. Russo, "History of Cannabis," 1614–1648; Dennis Kuo and Kathy D. Schlecht, "Hua Tuo and Mafeisan," *Journal of Anesthesia History* (2013): 52.
4. Mia Touw, "The Religious and Medicinal Uses of Cannabis in China, India and Tibet," *Journal of Psychoactive Drugs* 13, no. 1 (1981): 23–34; Natasha R. Ryz, David J. Remillard, and Ethan B. Russo, "Cannabis Roots: A Traditional Therapy with Future Potential for Treating Inflammation and Pain," *Cannabis and Cannabinoid Research* 2, no. 1 (2017): 210–216.
5. Antonio Walso Zuardi, "History of Cannabis as a Medicine: A Review," *Brazilian Journal of Psychiatry* 28, no. 2 (2006): 154.
6. Ethan B. Russo, "History of Cannabis and Its Preparations in Saga, Science, and Sobriquet," *Chemistry & Biodiversity* 4, no. 8 (2007): 1636.
7. Pisanti, "Medical Cannabis," 8342–8351.
8. Pisanti, "Medical Cannabis."
9. Russo, "History of Cannabis."
10. Pisanti, "Medical Cannabis."
11. Russo, "History of Cannabis."
12. Pisanti, "Medical Cannabis."
13. https://www.ancient-origins.net/news-history-archaeology/did-ancient-siberian-princess-use-cannabis-cope-breast-cancer-002207.
14. https://siberiantimes.com/other/others/features/tattooed-2500-year-old-siberian-princess-to-be-reburied/.
15. https://www.jewishboston.com/am-yisrael-high-cannabis-in-jewish-tradition/.
16. Pisanti, "Medical Cannabis."
17. Raphael Mechoulam, ed., *Cannabinoids as Therapeutic Agents* (Boca Raton, FL: CRC Press, 2019), 3.
18. http://antiquecannabisbook.com/chap2B/Greco_Roman/Pliny.htm, Book 20, 298.
19. Pisanti, "Medical Cannabis."
20. Pisanti, "Medical Cannabis."
21. Mechoulam, *Cannabinoids as Therapeutic Agents.*
22. Abel, *Marihuana.*
23. Pisanti, "Medical Cannabis."
24. Ethan Russo, "Hemp for Headache: An In-Depth Historical and Scientific Review of Cannabis in Migraine Treatment," *Journal of Cannabis Therapeutics* 1, no. 2 (2001): 29.
25. Pisanti, "Medical Cannabis."
26. http://www.complete-herbal.com/culpepper/hemp.htm.
27. Pisanti, "Medical Cannabis."
28. Simona Pisanti and Maurizio Bifulco, "Modern History of Medical Cannabis: From Widespread Use to Prohibitionism and Back," *Trends in Pharmacological Sciences* 38, no. 3 (2017): 195–198.

29. Mechoulam, *Cannabinoids as Therapeutic Agents.*
30. https://www.civilized.life/articles/prohibitionists-napoleon-bonaparte/.
31. Mechoulam, *Cannabinoids as Therapeutic Agents.*
32. B. Warf, "High Points: An Historical Geography of Cannabis," *Geographical Review* 104, no. 4 (2014): 414–438.
33. Mechoulam, *Cannabinoids as Therapeutic Agents,* 10–11.
34. Russo, "History of Cannabis."
35. https://publications.parliament.uk/pa/ld199798/ldselect/ldsctech/151/15103.htm.
36. https://publications.parliament.uk/pa/ld199798/ldselect/ldsctech/151/15103.htm.
37. Michael Aldrich, "History of Therapeutic Cannabis," in *Cannabis in Medical Practice* (Jefferson, NC: Mc Farland, 1997), 35–55.
38. Aldrich, "History of Therapeutic Cannabis."
39. Zuardi, "History of Cannabis," 153–157; Tod H. Mikuriya, "Marijuana in Medicine: Past, Present and Future," *California Medicine* 110, no. 1 (1969): 34–40.
40. Mechoulam, *Cannabinoids as Therapeutic Agents.*
41. Zuardi, "History of Cannabis."
42. Mikuriya, "Marijuana in Medicine."
43. Beth Wiese and Adrianne R. Wilson-Poe, "Emerging Evidence for Cannabis' Role in Opioid Use Disorder," *Cannabis and Cannabinoid Research* 3, no. 1 (2018): 179–189.
44. Zuardi, "History of Cannabis."
45. Mikuriya, "Marijuana in Medicine."
46. Mikuriya, "Marijuana in Medicine."
47. Isaac Campos, "Mexicans and the Origins of Marijuana Prohibition in the United States: A Reassessment," *The Social History of Alcohol and Drugs* 32, no. 1 (2018): 6–37.
48. Abel, *Marihuana.*
49. Abel, *Marihuana.*
50. http://www.druglibrary.org/schaffer/library/mj_outlawed.htm.
51. http://www.druglibrary.org/schaffer/history/casey1.htm.
52. Abel, *Marihuana.*
53. http://thevintagecameo.com/2014/01/la-fiesta-de-santa-barbara-1935/.
54. Abel, *Marihuana.*
55. David Bewley-Taylor, Tom Blickman, and Martin Jelsma, "The Rise and Decline of Cannabis Prohibition—The History of Cannabis in the UN Drug Control System and Options for Reform" (Amsterdam/Swansea: Global Drugs Policy Observatory Project/Transnational Institute, 2014).
56. M. Eddy, "Medical Marijuana: Review and Analysis of Federal and State Policies," Congressional Research Service, Library of Congress, 2007.
57. Bewley-Taylor, "The Rise and Decline of Cannabis Prohibition," 13–14.
58. "Report of the Committee on Legislative Activities," *JAMA* 108 (1937): 2214–2215, quoted in Todd Mikuriya, *Marijuana: Medical Papers* (Oakland, CA:

Medi-Comp Press, 1973), xiii–xxvii; https://www.druglibrary.net/schaffer/hemp/medical/medpaper.htm.

59. http://www.druglibrary.org/schaffer/hemp/taxact/mjtaxact.htm.
60. Edward M. Brecher, "The Consumers Union Report on Licit and Illicit Drugs," *Consumer Reports Magazine* (1972), chapter 56.
61. Fiorello LaGuardia and E. Corwin, "The Laguardia Committee Report New York, USA (1944)," https://www.druglibrary.org/schaffer/Library/studies/lag/lagmenu.htm.
62. Peat, Marwick, Mitchell and Co. and United States of America, "Marijuana—A Study of State Policies and Penalties" (1977). https://www.ncjrs.gov/pdffiles1/Digitization/43880NCJRS.pdf.
63. Peat, Marwick, "Marijuana—A Study of State Policies and Penalties."
64. https://www.csdp.org/research/nixonpot.txt.
65. https://www.cga.ct.gov/2010/rpt/2010-r-0204.htm.
66. Kasey C. Phillips, "Drug War Madness: A Call for Consistency Amidst the Conflict," *Chapman Law Review* 13 (2009): 645.
67. https://timesmachine.nytimes.com/timesmachine/1975/10/05/91188745.html?pageNumber=59.
68. https://www.fordlibrarymuseum.gov/library/document/0126/1489799.pdf.
69. https://www.history.com/topics/crime/the-war-on-drugs.
70. https://www.nytimes.com/1989/09/06/us/text-of-president-s-speech-on-national-drug-control-strategy.html.
71. https://www.justice.gov/archive/dag/pubdoc/Drug_Final.pdf.
72. https://www.sentencingproject.org/wp-content/uploads/2020/08/Trends-in-US-Corrections.pdf.
73. https://www.naacp.org/criminal-justice-fact-sheet/.
74. https://ucr.fbi.gov/crime-in-the-u.s/2000/00sec4.pdf.
75. https://harpers.org/archive/2016/04/legalize-it-all/.
76. Raphael Mechoulam, "Conversation with Raphael Mechoulam," *Addiction* 102, no. 6 (2007): 887–889.
77. Mechoulam, "Conversation with Raphael Mechoulam," 888.
78. https://medicalmarijuana.procon.org/legal-medical-marijuana-states-and-dc/.
79. https://law.emory.edu/ecgar/_documents/volumes/5/1/pickle.pdf.
80. https://www.forbes.com/sites/tomangell/2018/02/23/senator-calls-out-big-pharma-for-opposing-legal-marijuana/#ac77b511bac4.
81. https://law.emory.edu/ecgar/_documents/volumes/5/1/pickle.pdf.
82. Eric P. Baron et al., "Patterns of Medicinal Cannabis Use, Strain Analysis, and Substitution Effect among Patients with Migraine, Headache, Arthritis, and Chronic Pain in a Medicinal Cannabis Cohort," *The Journal of Headache and Pain* 19, no. 1 (2018): 1–28.
83. https://fas.org/sgp/crs/misc/R44742.pdf.
84. https://www.fda.gov/news-events/press-announcements/statement-fda-commissioner-scott-gottlieb-md-new-steps-advance-agencys-continued-evaluation.

85. Hongying Dai and Kimber P. Richter, "A National Survey of Marijuana Use among US Adults with Medical Conditions, 2016–2017," *JAMA Network Open* 2, no. 9 (2019): e1911936–e1911936.
86. Lindsey M. Philpot, Jon O. Ebbert, and Ryan T. Hurt, "A Survey of the Attitudes, Beliefs and Knowledge about Medical Cannabis among Primary Care Providers," *BMC Family Practice* 20, no. 1 (2019): 1–7.
87. https://www.latimes.com/world-nation/story/2020-10-12/mexico-is-poised-to-become-the-biggest-legal-marijuana-market-in-the-world-the-big-question-who-will-benefit?_amp=true.

CHAPTER 2: CANNABIS CLARIFIED

1. Caroline A. MacCallum and Ethan B. Russo, "Practical Considerations in Medical Cannabis Administration and Dosing," *European Journal of Internal Medicine* 49 (2018): 12–19.
2. https://pubchem.ncbi.nlm.nih.gov/compound/Tetrahydrocannabivarin.
3. https://pubchem.ncbi.nlm.nih.gov/compound/Tetrahydrocannabivarin.
4. Khalid A. Jadoon et al., "Efficacy and Safety of Cannabidiol and Tetrahydrocannabivarin on Glycemic and Lipid Parameters in Patients with Type 2 Diabetes: A Randomized, Double-Blind, Placebo-Controlled, Parallel Group Pilot Study," *Diabetes Care* 39, no. 10 (2016): 1777–1786.
5. Amos Abioye et al., "Δ9-Tetrahydrocannabivarin (THCV): A Commentary on Potential Therapeutic Benefit for the Management of Obesity and Diabetes," *Journal of Cannabis Research* 2, no. 1 (2020): 1–6.
6. Isabel Espadas et al., "Beneficial Effects of the Phytocannabinoid Δ9-THCV in L-DOPA-induced Dyskinesia in Parkinson's Disease," *Neurobiology of Disease* 141 (2020): 104892.
7. https://www.cancer.gov/publications/dictionaries/cancer-drug/def/delta-8-tetrahydrocannabinol?redirect=true.
8. https://www.dea.gov/sites/default/files/2020-04/Drugs%20of%20Abuse%202020-Web%20Version-508%20compliant-4-24-20_0.pdf.
9. Email message to Joan Liebmann-Smith, May 10, 2021.
10. Daniele Piomelli and Ethan B. Russo. "The Cannabis Sativa Versus Cannabis Indica Debate: An Interview with Ethan Russo, MD," *Cannabis and Cannabinoid Research* 1, no. 1 (2016): 44–46.
11. Rachel Knox, email message to board members of DFCR.org, July 23, 2020.
12. Joshua A. Hartsel et al., "Cannabis Sativa and Hemp," in *Nutraceuticals* (Cambridge, MA: Academic Press, 2016), 735–754; Zaid Maayah et al., "The Molecular Mechanisms That Underpin the Biological Benefits of Full-Spectrum Cannabis Extract in the Treatment of Neuropathic Pain and Inflammation," *Biochimica et Biophysica Acta (BBA)—Molecular Basis of Disease* 1866, no. 7 (2020): 165771; Eric P. Baron, "Medicinal Properties of Cannabinoids, Terpenes, and Flavonoids in Cannabis, and Benefits in Migraine, Headache, and Pain: An Update on Current Evidence and Cannabis Science," *Headache: The Journal of Head and Face Pain* 58, no. 7 (2018): 1139–1186.

13. Martin A. Lee, "The Discovery of the Endocannabinoid System," *The Prop* 215 (2012): 1. https://www.beyondthc.com/wp-content/uploads/2012/07/eCBSystemLee.pdf.
14. Raphael Mechoulam and Linda A. Parker, "The Endocannabinoid System and the Brain," *Annual Review of Psychology* 64 (2013): 21–47.
15. Mechoulam and Parker, "The Endocannabinoid System and the Brain."
16. https://www.projectcbd.org/science/cbd-clinical-endocannabinoid-deficiency.
17. Donald I. Abrams, "The Therapeutic Effects of Cannabis and Cannabinoids: An Update from the National Academies of Sciences, Engineering and Medicine Report," *European Journal of Internal Medicine* 49 (2018): 7–11.
18. Judith K. Booth and Jörg Bohlmann, "Terpenes in Cannabis Sativa—From Plant Genome to Humans," *Plant Science* 284 (2019): 67–72.
19. Lumír Ondřej Hanuš and Yotam Hod, "Terpenes/Terpenoids in Cannabis: Are They Important?," *Medical Cannabis and Cannabinoids* 3, no. 1 (2020): 33.
20. Ethan B. Russo, "Taming THC: Potential Cannabis Synergy and Phytocannabinoid-Terpenoid Entourage Effects," *British Journal of Pharmacology* 163, no. 7 (2011): 1344–1364; Hartsel, "Cannabis Sativa and Hemp"; Hanuš and Hod, "Terpenes/Terpenoids in Cannabis," 25–60; Baron, "Medicinal Properties of Cannabinoids"; Maayah, "The Molecular Mechanisms"; Xiao Yu et al., "D-limonene Exhibits Antitumor Activity by Inducing Autophagy and Apoptosis in Lung Cancer," *OncoTargets and Therapy* 11 (2018): 1833.
21. Hanuš and Hod, "Terpenes/Terpenoids in Cannabis."
22. https://www.webmd.com/cancer/rick-simpson-oil-for-cancer-overview#1.
23. National Academies of Sciences, Engineering, and Medicine, "The Health Effects of Cannabis and Cannabinoids: The Current State of Evidence and Recommendations for Research" (2017), https://www.nap.edu/catalog/24625/the-health-effects-of-cannabis-and-cannabinoids-the-current-state.
24. Abrams, "The Therapeutic Effects of Cannabis and Cannabinoids," 1.
25. Robert L. Page et al., "Medical Marijuana, Recreational Cannabis, and Cardiovascular Health: A Scientific Statement from the American Heart Association," *Circulation* 142, no. 10 (2020): e131–e152.
26. Kevin F. Boehnke et al., "Qualifying Conditions of Medical Cannabis License Holders in the United States," *Health Affairs* 38, no. 2 (2019): 295–302.
27. Kevin M. Takakuwa et al., "Education, Knowledge, and Practice Characteristics of Cannabis Physicians: A Survey of the Society of Cannabis Clinicians," *Cannabis and Cannabinoid Research* 6, no. 1 (2021): 58–65.
28. Beatriz H. Carlini, Sharon B. Garrett, and Gregory T. Carter, "Medicinal Cannabis: A Survey among Health Care Providers in Washington State," *American Journal of Hospice and Palliative Medicine* 34, no. 1 (2017): 85–91; Lindsey M. Philpot, Jon O. Ebbert, and Ryan T. Hurt, "A Survey of the Attitudes, Beliefs and Knowledge about Medical Cannabis among Primary Care Providers," *BMC Family Practice* 20, no. 1 (2019): 1–7.

29. Cayley Russell et al., "Routes of Administration for Cannabis Use—Basic Prevalence and Related Health Outcomes: A Scoping Review and Synthesis," *International Journal of Drug Policy* 52 (2018): 87–96.
30. National Academies of Sciences, "The Health Effects of Cannabis and Cannabinoids"; James Jett et al., "Cannabis Use, Lung Cancer, and Related Issues," *Journal of Thoracic Oncology* 13, no. 4 (2018): 480–487.
31. https://www.fda.gov/consumers/consumer-updates/what-you-need-know-and-what-were-working-find-out-about-products-containing-cannabis-or-cannabis.
32. Keith A. Sharkey, Nissar A. Darmani, and Linda A. Parker, "Regulation of Nausea and Vomiting by Cannabinoids and the Endocannabinoid System," *European Journal of Pharmacology* 722 (2014): 134–146.
33. Cecilia J. Sorensen et al., "Cannabinoid Hyperemesis Syndrome: Diagnosis, Pathophysiology, and Treatment—A Systematic Review," *Journal of Medical Toxicology* 13, no. 1 (2017): 71–87.
34. Sharkey, "Regulation of Nausea."
35. Xibei Liu, Angela Villamagna, and Ji Yoo, "The Importance of Recognizing Cannabinoid Hyperemesis Syndrome from Synthetic Marijuana Use," *Journal of Medical Toxicology* 13, no. 2 (2017): 199–200.
36. Page, "Medical Marijuana."
37. https://www.cdc.gov/marijuana/faqs/overdose-bad-reaction.html.
38. Daniel J. Corsi et al., "Association between Self-Reported Prenatal Cannabis Use and Maternal, Perinatal, and Neonatal Outcomes," *JAMA* 322, no. 2 (2019): 145–152; Sabrina Luke, Jennifer Hutcheon, and Tamil Kendall, "Cannabis Use in Pregnancy in British Columbia and Selected Birth Outcomes," *Journal of Obstetrics and Gynaecology Canada* 41, no. 9 (2019): 1311–1317; Shayna N. Conner et al., "Maternal Marijuana Use and Adverse Neonatal Outcomes," *Obstetrics & Gynecology* 128, no. 4 (2016): 713–723.
39. https://www.acog.org/-/media/project/acog/acogorg/clinical/files/committee-opinion/articles/2017/10/marijuana-use-during-pregnancy-and-lactation.pdf.
40. https://www.aappublications.org/news/aapnewsmag/2018/08/27/marijuana082718.full.pdf.
41. https://www.cdc.gov/marijuana/pdf/marijuana-pregnancy-508.pdf.
42. Erich Goode, *The Marijuana Smokers* (New York: Basic Books, 2004), 185–190.
43. https://ucr.fbi.gov/crime-in-the-u.s/2000/00sec4.pdf.
44. American Psychiatric Association, *Diagnostic and Statistical Manual of Mental Disorders*, 5th ed. (Washington, DC: American Psychiatric Press, 2015), 485. https://cdn.website-editor.net/30f11123991548a0af708722d458e476/files/uploaded/DSM%2520V.pdf.
45. https://www.drugabuse.gov/publications/research-reports/marijuana/marijuana-addictive.
46. https://www.ncbi.nlm.nih.gov/pmc/articles/PMC4444130/.

47. Valentina Gritsenko et al., "Religion in Russia: Its Impact on University Student Medical Cannabis Attitudes and Beliefs," *Complementary Therapies in Medicine* 54 (2020): 102546.
48. Robert A. Mikos and Cindy D. Kam, "Has the 'M' Word Been Framed? Marijuana, Cannabis, and Public Opinion," *PLOS ONE* 14, no. 10 (2019): 8.
49. I. Rezik, "Cannabinoids-Based Medicine as a Pivotal Model for Personalized Integrative Care," in A. Aran et al., 4th International Medical Cannabis Conference (CannX 2019), Tel Aviv, Israel, September 9–10, 2019, 13, https://www.karger.com/Article/Pdf/502323.
50. Rachel Knox, email message to board members of DFCR.org, July 23, 2020.
51. Sharad Goyal, Sindhu Kubendran, Mikhail Kogan, and Yuan J. Rao, "High Expectations: The Landscape of Clinical Trials of Medical Marijuana in Oncology," *Complementary Therapies in Medicine* 49 (2020): 102336.
52. https://www.federalregister.gov/public-inspection/2020-27999/controls-to-enhance-the-cultivation-of-marihuana-for-research-in-the-united-states.
53. https://www.dea.gov/stories/2021/2021-05/2021-05-14/dea-continues-prioritize-efforts-expand-access-marijuana-research.
54. National Academies of Sciences, "The Health Effects of Cannabis and Cannabinoids."
55. Page, "Medical Marijuana."
56. Page, "Medical Marijuana," e148.

CHAPTER 3: FINDING THE RIGHT ROUTE

1. Ethan B. Russo, "History of Cannabis and Its Preparations in Saga, Science, and Sobriquet," *Chemistry & Biodiversity* 4, no. 8 (2007): 1614–1648.
2. Meng Ren et al., "The Origins of Cannabis Smoking: Chemical Residue Evidence from the First Millennium BCE in the Pamirs," *Science Advances* 5, no. 6 (2019): eaaw1391.
3. Mallory Loflin and Mitch Earleywine, "No Smoke, No Fire: What the Initial Literature Suggests Regarding Vapourized Cannabis and Respiratory Risk," *Canadian Journal of Respiratory Therapy: CJRT=Revue Canadienne de la Therapie Respiratoire: RCTR* 51, no. 1 (2015): 7.
4. Cayley Russell et al., "Routes of Administration for Cannabis Use—Basic Prevalence and Related Health Outcomes: A Scoping Review and Synthesis," *International Journal of Drug Policy* 52 (2018): 87–96.
5. James Jett et al., "Cannabis Use, Lung Cancer, and Related Issues," *Journal of Thoracic Oncology* 13, no. 4 (2018): 480–487.
6. https://www.cdc.gov/mmwr/volumes/69/wr/mm6925a5.htm.
7. https://www.cdc.gov/mmwr/volumes/69/wr/mm6925a5.htm.
8. https://www.cdph.ca.gov/Programs/CCDPHP/SiteAssets/Pages/EVALI-Weekly-Public-Report/CDPH%20Advisory%20EVALI%20Case%20Definition%20Update_May%209,%202020.pdf, 4.
9. Jett, "Cannabis Use, Lung Cancer."

10. Robert L. Page et al., "Medical Marijuana, Recreational Cannabis, and Cardiovascular Health: A Scientific Statement from the American Heart Association," *Circulation* 142, no. 10 (2020): e131–e152.
11. Francisco Pastor et al., "Therapeutic Cannabis and COVID-19: Between Opportunism and Infoxication" ("Cannabis Terapéutico y COVID-19: Entre el Oportunismo y la Infoxicación"), *Adicciones* 32, no. 3 (2020): 167–172.
12. Sherry Yafai and Stuart Etengoff, "The Case for Cannabis: Advising Cannabis Users about COVID-19," *Emergency Medicine News* 42, no. 5B (2020). https://journals.lww.com/em-news/fulltext/2020/05201/the_case_for_cannabis__advising__cannabis__users.4.aspx.
13. Yafai and Etengoff, "The Case for Cannabis."
14. Veronica Stahl and Kumar Vasudevan, "Comparison of Efficacy of Cannabinoids versus Commercial Oral Care Products in Reducing Bacterial Content from Dental Plaque: A Preliminary Observation," *Cureus* 12, no. 1 (2020).
15. Kumar Vasudevan and Veronica Stahl, "Cannabinoids-Infused Mouthwash Products Are as Effective as Chlorhexidine on Inhibition of Total-Culturable Bacterial Content in Dental Plaque Samples," *Journal of Cannabis Research* 2, no. 1 (2020): 1–9.
16. John R. Richards, Nishelle E. Smith, and Aimee K. Moulin, "Unintentional Cannabis Ingestion in Children: A Systematic Review," *The Journal of Pediatrics* 190 (2017): 142–152.
17. Andrew A. Monte, Richard D. Zane, and Kennon J. Heard, "The Implications of Marijuana Legalization in Colorado," *JAMA* 313, no. 3 (2015): 241–242.
18. Daniel G. Barrus et al., "Tasty THC: Promises and Challenges of Cannabis Edibles," *Methods Report* (Research Triangle Park, NC: RTI Press, 2016).
19. https://www.ift.org/news-and-publications/food-technology-magazine/issues/2019/february/features/cannabis-edibles.
20. https://www.alliedmarketresearch.com/cbd-skin-care-market.
21. Carmen Del Río et al., "The Endocannabinoid System of the Skin: A Potential Approach for the Treatment of Skin Disorders," *Biochemical Pharmacology* 157 (2018): 122–133.
22. Raphael Mechoulam, ed., *Cannabinoids as Therapeutic Agents* (Boca Raton, FL: CRC Press, 2019).
23. John W. Farlow, "On the Use of Belladonna and Cannabis Indica by the Rectum in Gynecological Practice," *The Boston Medical and Surgical Journal* 120, no. 21 (1889): 507–509.

CHAPTER 4: ACHES AND PAINS

1. https://allauthor.com/quotes/113864/.
2. Ji-Yeun Park and Li-Tzy Wu, "Prevalence, Reasons, Perceived Effects, and Correlates of Medical Marijuana Use: A Review," *Drug and Alcohol Dependence* 177 (2017): 1–13.
3. https://www.nap.edu/catalog/24625/the-health-effects-of-cannabis-and-cannabinoids-the-current-state.

4. James Dahlhamer et al., "Prevalence of Chronic Pain and High-Impact Chronic Pain among Adults—United States, 2016," *Morbidity and Mortality Weekly Report* 67, no. 36 (2018): 1001.
5. Darrell J. Gaskin and Patrick Richard, "The Economic Costs of Pain in the United States," *The Journal of Pain* 13, no. 8 (2012): 715–724.
6. https://www.cdc.gov/drugoverdose/data/statedeaths.html.
7. https://www.ajmc.com/journals/issue/2020/2020-vol26-n7/the-escalation-of-the-opioid-epidemic-due-to-covid19-and-resulting-lessons-about-treatment-alternatives.
8. https://www.samhsa.gov/data/sites/default/files/reports/rpt29393/2019NSDUHFFRPDFWHTML/2019NSDUHFFR1PDFW090120.pdf.
9. E. Alfonso Romero-Sandoval et al., "Cannabis for Chronic Pain: Challenges and Considerations," *Pharmacotherapy: The Journal of Human Pharmacology and Drug Therapy* 38, no. 6 (2018): 651–662.
10. National Academies of Sciences, Engineering, and Medicine, "The Health Effects of Cannabis and Cannabinoids: The Current State of Evidence and Recommendations for Research" (2017), 13, https://www.nap.edu/read/24625/chapter/2#13.
11. Nicholas Culpeper, *Culpeper's Complete Herbal: A Book of Natural Remedies for Ancient Ills* (1653), reprint (Wordsworth Editions, 1995), http://antiquecannabisbook.com/chap1/Witchs.htm.
12. Jayesh R. Parmar, Benjamin D. Forrest, and Robert A. Freeman, "Medical Marijuana Patient Counseling Points for Health Care Professionals Based on Trends in the Medical Uses, Efficacy, and Adverse Effects of Cannabis-Based Pharmaceutical Drugs," *Research in Social and Administrative Pharmacy* 12, no. 4 (2016): 638–654.
13. Romero-Sandoval, "Cannabis for Chronic Pain."
14. Romero-Sandoval, "Cannabis for Chronic Pain," 4.
15. https://www.rheumatoidarthritis.org/ra/ra-vs-oa/.
16. Richard J. Miller and Rachel E. Miller, "Is Cannabis an Effective Treatment for Joint Pain?," *Clinical and Experimental Rheumatology* 35, no. 5 (2017): 59–67.
17. https://creakyjoints.org/eular-2019/medical-marijuana-cbd-usage-arthritis-patients-study/.
18. https://creakyjoints.org/eular-2019/medical-marijuana-cbd-usage-arthritis-patients-study/.
19. Kelly Gavigan et al., "Patients' Perception and Use of Medical Marijuana," *Annals of the Rheumatic Diseases* 78, Suppl 2 (2019): 617–618.
20. https://migraineresearchfoundation.org/about-migraine/migraine-facts/.
21. Carrie Cuttler et al., "Short- and Long-Term Effects of Cannabis on Headache and Migraine," *The Journal of Pain* 21, no. 5–6 (2020): 722–730.
22. Eric P. Baron et al., "Patterns of Medicinal Cannabis Use, Strain Analysis, and Substitution Effect among Patients with Migraine, Headache, Arthritis,

and Chronic Pain in a Medicinal Cannabis Cohort," *The Journal of Headache and Pain* 19, no. 1 (2018): 1–28.

23. Baron, "Patterns of Medicinal Cannabis Use."
24. Ellen Feldman, "Cannabis in the Treatment of Headache and Migraine," *Integrative Medicine Alert* 23, no. 4 (2020).
25. Cuttler, "Short- and Long-Term Effects"; Laszlo Mechtler et al., "Medical Cannabis for Chronic Migraine: A Retrospective Review," *Neurology* 92, Suppl 15 (2019): P3. 10–015.
26. Joshua Aviram et al., "Migraine Frequency Decrease Following Prolonged Medical Cannabis Treatment: A Cross-Sectional Study," *Brain Sciences* 10, no. 6 (2020): 360.
27. Mechtler, "Medical Cannabis for Chronic Migraine"; Baron, "Patterns of Medicinal Cannabis Use."
28. Kevin P. Hill, "Medical Marijuana for Treatment of Chronic Pain and Other Medical and Psychiatric Problems: A Clinical Review," *JAMA* 313, no. 24 (2015): 2474.
29. Romero-Sandoval, "Cannabis for Chronic Pain."
30. Romero-Sandoval, "Cannabis for Chronic Pain."
31. http://www.fmaware.org/about-fibromyalgia/prevalence/.
32. http://www.fmaware.org/about-fibromyalgia/prevalence/.
33. Ethan B. Russo, "Clinical Endocannabinoid Deficiency Reconsidered: Current Research Supports the Theory in Migraine, Fibromyalgia, Irritable Bowel, and Other Treatment-Resistant Syndromes," *Cannabis and Cannabinoid Research* 1, no. 1 (2016): 154–165.
34. Roie Tzadok and Jacob N. Ablin, "Current and Emerging Pharmacotherapy for Fibromyalgia," *Pain Research and Management* 10 (2020): 1–9.
35. Pat Anson, "Marijuana Rated Most Effective for Treating Fibromyalgia," *National Pain Foundation* (2014), http://www.medicalmarijuana.eu/survey-shows-fibromyalgia-patients-find-cannabis-effective-treatment/.
36. Anson, "Marijuana Rated Most Effective."
37. George Habib and Irit Avisar, "The Consumption of Cannabis by Fibromyalgia Patients in Israel," *Pain Research and Treatment* (2018).
38. Iftach Sagy et al., "Safety and Efficacy of Medical Cannabis in Fibromyalgia," *Journal of Clinical Medicine* 8, no. 6 (2019): 807.
39. Marco D. DiBonaventura et al., "The Prevalence of Probable Neuropathic Pain in the US: Results from a Multimodal General-Population Health Survey," *Journal of Pain Research* 10 (2017): 2525.
40. Luana Colloca et al., "Neuropathic Pain," *Nature Reviews Disease Primers* 3, no. 1 (2017): 1–19.
41. Donald I. Abrams et al., "Cannabis in Painful HIV-Associated Sensory Neuropathy: A Randomized Placebo-Controlled Trial," *Neurology* 68, no. 7 (2007): 515–521.
42. Romero-Sandoval, "Cannabis for Chronic Pain."

43. Simon Vulfsons, Amir Minerbi, and Tali Sahar, "Cannabis and Pain Treatment—A Review of the Clinical Utility and a Practical Approach in Light of Uncertainty," *Rambam Maimonides Medical Journal* 11, no. 1 (2020).
44. David J. Casarett, Jessica N. Beliveau, and Michelle S. Arbus, "Benefit of Tetrahydrocannabinol versus Cannabidiol for Common Palliative Care Symptoms," *Journal of Palliative Medicine* 22, no. 10 (2019): 1180–1184.
45. https://www.medicalnewstoday.com/articles/160253; https://www.cdc.gov/shingles/surveillance.html.
46. Ngoc Quan Phan et al., "Adjuvant Topical Therapy with a Cannabinoid Receptor Agonist in Facial Postherpetic Neuralgia," *JDDG: Journal der Deutschen Dermatologischen Gesellschaft* 8, no. 2 (2010): 88–91.
47. Karma Rabgay et al., "The Effects of Cannabis, Cannabinoids, and Their Administration Routes on Pain Control Efficacy and Safety: A Systematic Review and Network Meta-Analysis," *Journal of the American Pharmacists Association* 60, no. 1 (2020): 225–234.
48. Asfandyar Khan Niazi and Shaharyar Khan Niazi, "Mindfulness-Based Stress Reduction: A Non-Pharmacological Approach for Chronic Illnesses," *North American Journal of Medical Sciences* 3, no. 1 (2011): 20.
49. Willard C. Harrill, "Vaping during the COVID-19 Pandemic: NOT GOOD!!," *Laryngoscope Investigative Otolaryngology* 5, no. 3 (2020): 399.
50. Harrill, "Vaping during the COVID-19 Pandemic."
51. The Lancet Respiratory Medicine, "The EVALI Outbreak and Vaping in the COVID-19 Era," *The Lancet* (2020).
52. Robert L. Page et al., "Medical Marijuana, Recreational Cannabis, and Cardiovascular Health: A Scientific Statement from the American Heart Association," *Circulation* 142, no. 10 (2020): e131–e152.
53. Tory R. Spindle, Marcel O. Bonn-Miller, and Ryan Vandrey, "Changing Landscape of Cannabis: Novel Products, Formulations, and Methods of Administration," *Current Opinion in Psychology* 30 (2019): 98–102.
54. Natascia Bruni et al., "Cannabinoid Delivery Systems for Pain and Inflammation Treatment," *Molecules* 23, no. 10 (2018): 2478.
55. Xiaoxue Li et al., "The Effectiveness of Self-Directed Medical Cannabis Treatment for Pain," *Complementary Therapies in Medicine* 46 (2019): 123–130.
56. E. Alfonso Romero-Sandoval et al., "Peripherally Restricted Cannabinoids for the Treatment of Pain," *Pharmacotherapy: The Journal of Human Pharmacology and Drug Therapy* 35, no. 10 (2015): 917–925.
57. Simona Pisanti and Maurizio Bifulco, "Medical Cannabis: A Plurimillennial History of an Evergreen," *Journal of Cellular Physiology* 234, no. 6 (2019): 8342–8351.
58. Sara Ward, "Analgesic Efficacy of Single and Combined Minor Cannabinoids and Terpenes" (2020), https://grantome.com/grant/NIH/R01-AT010778-01.
59. https://virtual.painweek.org//2020/painweek/searchGlobal.asp?mode=posters&SearchQuery=cannabis.

60. https://virtual.painweek.org//2020/painweek/searchGlobal.asp?mode=posters&SearchQuery=cannabis.
61. F. Bache, *The Dispensatory of the United States of America*, vol. 1238, 6th ed. (Philadelphia: Grigg and Elliot, 1845).
62. Beth Wiese and Adrianne R. Wilson-Poe, "Emerging Evidence for Cannabis' Role in Opioid Use Disorder," *Cannabis and Cannabinoid Research* 3, no. 1 (2018): 179–189.
63. Ramin Safakish et al., "Medical Cannabis for the Management of Pain and Quality of Life in Chronic Pain Patients: A Prospective Observational Study," *Pain Medicine* 21, no. 11 (2020): 3073–3086.
64. https://www.nap.edu/catalog/24625/the-health-effects-of-cannabis-and-cannabinoids-the-current-state; Romero-Sandoval, "Cannabis for Chronic Pain"; Eric P. Baron et al., "Patterns of Medicinal Cannabis Use, Strain Analysis, and Substitution Effect among Patients with Migraine, Headache, Arthritis, and Chronic Pain in a Medicinal Cannabis Cohort," *The Journal of Headache and Pain* 19, no. 1 (2018): 1–28.
65. Baron et al., "Patterns of Medicinal Cannabis Use."

CHAPTER 5: SLEEP AND MOOD

1. Jacqueline M. Doremus, Sarah S. Stith, and Jacob M. Vigil, "Using Recreational Cannabis to Treat Insomnia: Evidence from Over-the-Counter Sleep Aid Sales in Colorado," *Complementary Therapies in Medicine* 47 (2019): 4.
2. https://www.sleepassociation.org/about-sleep/sleep-statistics/; http://www.cdc.gov/mmwr/PDF/wk/mm6008.pdf.
3. https://www.ninds.nih.gov/Disorders/patient-caregiver-education/understanding-sleep#2.
4. James K. Walsh et al., "Nighttime Insomnia Symptoms and Perceived Health in the America Insomnia Survey (AIS)," *Sleep* 34, no. 8 (2011): 997–1011.
5. Doremus, "Using Recreational Cannabis."
6. Shelly L. Gray et al., "Cumulative Use of Strong Anticholinergics and Incident Dementia: A Prospective Cohort Study," *JAMA Internal Medicine* 175, no. 3 (2015): 401–407.
7. https://www.cdc.gov/nchs/data/databriefs/db127.pdf.
8. https://www.fda.gov/drugs/drug-safety-and-availability/fda-adds-boxed-warning-risk-serious-injuries-caused-sleepwalking-certain-prescription-insomnia.
9. https://www.drugabuse.gov/related-topics/trends-statistics/overdose-death-rates.
10. Daniel F. Kripke, Robert D. Langer, and Lawrence E. Kline, "Hypnotics' Association with Mortality or Cancer: A Matched Cohort Study," *BMJ Open* 2, no. 1 (2012).
11. Seockhoon Chung, Soyoung Youn, Kikyoung Yi, Boram Park, and Suyeon Lee, "Sleeping Pill Administration Time and Patient Subjective Satisfaction," *Journal of Clinical Sleep Medicine* 12, no. 1 (2016): 57–62.

12. Manfred Fankhauser, "Cannabis as Medicine in Europe in the 19th Century" (1869). https://abuse-drug.com/lib/Cannabis-Reader/chapter-1-cannabis-as-medicine-in-europe-in-the-19th-century.html.
13. Kimberly A. Babson, James Sottile, and Danielle Morabito, "Cannabis, Cannabinoids, and Sleep: A Review of the Literature," *Current Psychiatry Reports* 19, no. 4 (2017): 1–12.
14. Geneviève Lafaye et al., "Cannabidiol Affects Circadian Clock Core Complex and Its Regulation in Microglia Cells," *Addiction Biology* 24, no. 5 (2019): 921–934.
15. National Academies of Sciences, Engineering, and Medicine, "The Health Effects of Cannabis and Cannabinoids: The Current State of Evidence and Recommendations for Research" (2017), 123. https://www.nap.edu/catalog/24625/the-health-effects-of-cannabis-and-cannabinoids-the-current-state.
16. Babson, "Cannabis, Cannabinoids, and Sleep."
17. Babson, "Cannabis, Cannabinoids, and Sleep."
18. Brian J. Piper et al., "Substitution of Medical Cannabis for Pharmaceutical Agents for Pain, Anxiety, and Sleep," *Journal of Psychopharmacology* 31, no. 5 (2017): 569–575.
19. Jacob M. Vigil et al., "Effectiveness of Raw, Natural Medical Cannabis Flower for Treating Insomnia under Naturalistic Conditions," *Medicines* 5, no. 3 (2018): 75.
20. Marcus Bachhuber, Julia H. Arnsten, and Gwen Wurm, "Use of Cannabis to Relieve Pain and Promote Sleep by Customers at an Adult Use Dispensary," *Journal of Psychoactive Drugs* 51, no. 5 (2019): 400–404.
21. Kimberly A. Babson and Marcel O. Bonn-Miller, "Sleep Disturbances: Implications for Cannabis Use, Cannabis Use Cessation, and Cannabis Use Treatment," *Current Addiction Reports* 1, no. 2 (2014): 109–114.
22. W. Ley, "Observations on the Cannabis Indica, or Indian Hemp," *Provincial Medical Journal and Retrospect of the Medical Sciences* 5, no. 129 (1843): 487.
23. Babson and Bonn-Miller, "Sleep Disturbances."
24. https://adaa.org/understanding-anxiety/posttraumatic-stress-disorder-ptsd.
25. https://www.ptsd.va.gov/understand/related/nightmares.asp.
26. Emma Paintain and Simon Cassidy, "First-Line Therapy for Post-Traumatic Stress Disorder: A Systematic Review of Cognitive Behavioural Therapy and Psychodynamic Approaches," *Counselling and Psychotherapy Research* 18, no. 3 (2018): 237–250.
27. Mallory J. E. Loflin et al., "Cannabinoids as Therapeutic for PTSD," *Current Opinion in Psychology* 14 (2017): 78–83.
28. Kevin Betthauser, Jeffrey Pilz, and Laura E. Vollmer, "Use and Effects of Cannabinoids in Military Veterans with Posttraumatic Stress Disorder," *American Journal of Health-System Pharmacy* 72, no. 15 (2015): 1279–1284.
29. Loflin, "Cannabinoids as Therapeutic."

30. https://norml.org/blog/2020/03/12/house-veterans-affairs-committee-passes-multiple-marijuana-bills/.
31. https://www.statista.com/statistics/1105365/coronavirus-sales-surge-of-recreational-cannabis-by-day-us/.
32. Denise C. Vidot et al., "The COVID-19 Cannabis Health Study: Results from an Epidemiologic Assessment of Adults Who Use Cannabis for Medicinal Reasons in the United States," *Journal of Addictive Diseases* 39, no. 1 (2021): 26–36.
33. Jesse D. Kosiba, Stephen A. Maisto, and Joseph W. Ditre, "Patient-Reported Use of Medical Cannabis for Pain, Anxiety, and Depression Symptoms: Systematic Review and Meta-Analysis," *Social Science & Medicine* 233 (2019): 181–192.
34. Zach Walsh et al., "Medical Cannabis and Mental Health: A Guided Systematic Review," *Clinical Psychology Review* 51 (2017): 15–29; Jasmine Turna, Beth Patterson, and Michael Van Ameringen, "Is Cannabis Treatment for Anxiety, Mood, and Related Disorders Ready for Prime Time?," *Depression and Anxiety* 34, no. 11 (2017): 1006–1017; Piper, "Substitution of Medical Cannabis"; Ji-Yeun Park and Li-Tzy Wu, "Prevalence, Reasons, Perceived Effects, and Correlates of Medical Marijuana Use: A Review," *Drug and Alcohol Dependence* 177 (2017): 1–13.
35. Jesse D. Kosiba, Stephen A. Maisto, and Joseph W. Ditre, "Patient-Reported Use of Medical Cannabis for Pain, Anxiety, and Depression Symptoms: Systematic Review and Meta-Analysis," *Social Science & Medicine* 233 (2019): 181–192.
36. Turna et al., "Is Cannabis Treatment for Anxiety?"
37. National Academies of Sciences, Engineering, and Medicine, "The Health Effects of Cannabis and Cannabinoids: The Current State of Evidence and Recommendations for Research" (2017). https://www.ncbi.nlm.nih.gov/books/NBK425767/.
38. Turna et al., "Is Cannabis Treatment for Anxiety?"
39. Turna et al., "Is Cannabis Treatment for Anxiety?"; Loflin, "Cannabinoids as Therapeutic."
40. Loflin, "Cannabinoids as Therapeutic."
41. Piper, "Substitution of Medical Cannabis"; James M. Corroon Jr., Laurie K. Mischley, and Michelle Sexton, "Cannabis as a Substitute for Prescription Drugs—A Cross-Sectional Study," *Journal of Pain Research* 10 (2017): 989; Helen Nunberg, Beau Kilmer, Rosalie Liccardo Pacula, and James R. Burgdorf, "An Analysis of Applicants Presenting to a Medical Marijuana Specialty Practice in California," *Journal of Drug Policy Analysis* 4, no. 1 (2011): 1.
42. Philippe Lucas and Zach Walsh, "Medical Cannabis Access, Use, and Substitution for Prescription Opioids and Other Substances: A Survey of Authorized Medical Cannabis Patients," *International Journal of Drug Policy* 42 (2017): 30–35.

43. Carrie Cuttler, Alexander Spradlin, and Ryan J. McLaughlin, "A Naturalistic Examination of the Perceived Effects of Cannabis on Negative Affect," *Journal of Affective Disorders* 235 (2018): 198–205.
44. Xiaoxue Li et al., "Focus: Plant-Based Medicine and Pharmacology: The Effectiveness of Cannabis Flower for Immediate Relief from Symptoms of Depression," *The Yale Journal of Biology and Medicine* 93, no. 2 (2020): 251–264.
45. John Clendinning, "Observations on the Medicinal Properties of the Cannabis Sativa of India," *Medico-Chirurgical Transactions* 26 (1843): 209.
46. Li et al., "Focus," 259.

CHAPTER 6: GASTROINTESTINAL DISORDERS

1. Antonio Waldo Zuardi, "History of Cannabis as a Medicine: A Review," *Brazilian Journal of Psychiatry* 28, no. 2 (2006): 153–157.
2. Raphael Mechoulam, ed., *Cannabinoids as Therapeutic Agents* (Boca Raton, FL: CRC Press, 2019), 22.
3. Sean D. Delshad et al., "Prevalence of Gastroesophageal Reflux Disease and Proton Pump Inhibitor-Refractory Symptoms," *Gastroenterology* 158, no. 5 (2020): 1250–1261; Erica Cohen et al., "GERD Symptoms in the General Population: Prevalence and Severity versus Care-Seeking Patients," *Digestive Diseases and Sciences* 59, no. 10 (2014): 2488–2496.
4. Maxwell M. Chait, "Gastroesophageal Reflux Disease: Important Considerations for the Older Patients," *World Journal of Gastrointestinal Endoscopy* 2, no. 12 (2010): 388.
5. https://www.mayoclinicproceedings.org/article/S0025-6196(17)30841-8/fulltext.
6. https://www.cdc.gov/media/releases/2015/p0225-clostridium-difficile.html.
7. https://www.iffgd.org/diet-treatments/antacids.html.
8. Jacqueline M. Doremus, Sarah S. Stith, and Jacob M. Vigil, "Off-Label Use of Recreational Cannabis: Acid Reflux in Colorado," *Economics Bulletin* 40, no. 1 (2020): 338–348.
9. Omar Abdel-Salam, "Gastric Acid Inhibitory and Gastric Protective Effects of Cannabis and Cannabinoids," *Asian Pacific Journal of Tropical Medicine* 9, no. 5 (2016): 413–419.
10. Doremus, "Off-Label Use."
11. https://www.aboutibs.org/facts-about-ibs.html.
12. https://gi.org/topics/irritable-bowel-syndrome/.
13. https://www.hopkinsmedicine.org/health/wellness-and-prevention/fodmap-diet-what-you-need-to-know.
14. Jessica L. Buono et al., "Economic Burden of Inadequate Symptom Control among US Commercially Insured Patients with Irritable Bowel Syndrome with Diarrhea," *Journal of Medical Economics* 20, no. 4 (2017): 353–362.
15. Ethan B. Russo, "Clinical Endocannabinoid Deficiency Reconsidered: Current Research Supports the Theory in Migraine, Fibromyalgia, Irritable

Bowel, and Other Treatment-Resistant Syndromes," *Cannabis and Cannabinoid Research* 1, no. 1 (2016): 154–165.

16. Ethan B. Russo, "History of Cannabis and Its Preparations in Saga, Science, and Sobriquet," *Chemistry & Biodiversity* 4, no. 8 (2007): 1614–1648.
17. Banny S. Wong et al., "Pharmacogenetic Trial of a Cannabinoid Agonist Shows Reduced Fasting Colonic Motility in Patients with Nonconstipated Irritable Bowel Syndrome," *Gastroenterology* 141, no. 5 (2011): 1638–1647.
18. Mikhail Kogan, ed., *Integrative Geriatric Medicine* (New York: Oxford University Press, 2017).
19. https://www.cdc.gov/mmwr/volumes/65/wr/mm6542a3.htm.
20. https://www.crohnscolitisfoundation.org/sites/default/files/2019-02/Updated%20IBD%20Factbook.pdf.
21. https://www.crohnscolitisfoundation.org/sites/default/files/legacy/assets/pdfs/surgery_brochure_final.pdf.
22. Silvio Danese et al., "Unmet Medical Needs in Ulcerative Colitis: An Expert Group Consensus," *Digestive Diseases* 37, no. 4 (2019): 266–283.
23. Meenakshi Bewtra and F. Reed Johnson, "Assessing Patient Preferences for Treatment Options and Process of Care in Inflammatory Bowel Disease: A Critical Review of Quantitative Data," *The Patient: Patient-Centered Outcomes Research* 6, no. 4 (2013): 241–255.
24. Orna Nitzan et al., "Clostridium Difficile and Inflammatory Bowel Disease: Role in Pathogenesis and Implications in Treatment," *World Journal of Gastroenterology: WJG* 19, no. 43 (2013): 7577.
25. Udayakumar Navaneethan, Preethi G. K. Venkatesh, and Bo Shen, "Clostridium Difficile Infection and Inflammatory Bowel Disease: Understanding the Evolving Relationship," *World Journal of Gastroenterology: WJG* 16, no. 39 (2010): 4892.
26. Jordan E. Axelrad, Simon Lichtiger, and Vijay Yajnik, "Inflammatory Bowel Disease and Cancer: The Role of Inflammation, Immunosuppression, and Cancer Treatment," *World Journal of Gastroenterology* 22, no. 20 (2016): 4794.
27. https://www.consumerreports.org/cro/2014/08/best-drugs-to-treat-inflammatory-bowel-disease/index.htm.
28. Chao Chen et al., "Real-world Pattern of Biologic Use in Patients with Inflammatory Bowel Disease: Treatment Persistence, Switching, and Importance of Concurrent Immunosuppressive Therapy," *Inflammatory Bowel Diseases* 25, no. 8 (2019): 1417–1427.
29. Steven C. Lin and Adam S. Cheifetz, "The Use of Complementary and Alternative Medicine in Patients with Inflammatory Bowel Disease," *Gastroenterology & Hepatology* 14, no. 7 (2018): 415; Melanie Kienzl, Martin Storr, and Rudolf Schicho, "Cannabinoids and Opioids in the Treatment of Inflammatory Bowel Diseases," *Clinical and Translational Gastroenterology* 11, no. 1 (2020).

30. Timna Naftali, "Is Cannabis of Potential Value as a Therapeutic for Inflammatory Bowel Disease?," 64, no. 10 (2019): 2696–2698.
31. Samiksha Pandey et al., "Endocannabinoid System in Irritable Bowel Syndrome and Cannabis as a Therapy," *Complementary Therapies in Medicine* 48 (2020): 102242.
32. Kienzl, "Cannabinoids and Opioids"; Abhilash Perisetti, Afrina Hossain Rimu, Salman Ali Khan, Pardeep Bansal, and Hemant Goyal, "Role of Cannabis in Inflammatory Bowel Diseases," *Annals of Gastroenterology* 33, no. 2 (2020): 134.
33. Martin Storr, Shane Devlin, Gilaad G. Kaplan, Remo Panaccione, and Christopher N. Andrews, "Cannabis Use Provides Symptom Relief in Patients with Inflammatory Bowel Disease but Is Associated with Worse Disease Prognosis in Patients with Crohn's Disease," *Inflammatory Bowel Diseases* 20, no. 3 (2014): 472–480.
34. Chimezie Mbachi et al., "Association between Cannabis Use and Complications Related to Crohn's Disease: A Retrospective Cohort Study," *Digestive Diseases and Sciences* 64, no. 10 (2019): 2939–2944.
35. Kienzl, "Cannabinoids and Opioids," 3–4.
36. Katherine E. MacDuffie et al., "Protection versus Progress: The Challenge of Research on Cannabis Use During Pregnancy," *Pediatrics* 146, Suppl 1 (2020): S93–S98.
37. MacDuffie et al., "Protection versus Progress."
38. Gideon Koren and Rana Cohen, "The Use of Cannabis for Hyperemesis Gravidarum (HG)," *Journal of Cannabis Research* 2, no. 1 (2020): 1–4; Judy C. Chang et al., "Beliefs and Attitudes Regarding Prenatal Marijuana Use: Perspectives of Pregnant Women Who Report Use," *Drug and Alcohol Dependence* 196 (2019): 14–20.
39. Daniel J. Corsi et al., "Association between Self-Reported Prenatal Cannabis Use and Maternal, Perinatal, and Neonatal Outcomes," *JAMA* 322, no. 2 (2019): 145–152; Sabrina Luke, Jennifer Hutcheon, and Tamil Kendall, "Cannabis Use in Pregnancy in British Columbia and Selected Birth Outcomes," *Journal of Obstetrics and Gynaecology Canada* 41, no. 9 (2019): 1311–1317; Shayna N. Conner et al., "Maternal Marijuana Use and Adverse Neonatal Outcomes," *Obstetrics & Gynecology* 128, no. 4 (2016): 713–723.
40. Conner et al., "Maternal Marijuana Use and Adverse Neonatal Outcomes."
41. MacDuffie et al., "Protection versus Progress."
42. MacDuffie et al., "Protection versus Progress."

CHAPTER 7: SKIN PROBLEMS

1. Lauren R. M. Eagleston et al., "Cannabinoids in Dermatology: A Scoping Review," *Dermatology Online Journal* 24, no. 6 (2018).
2. https://nationaleczema.org/warnings-for-topical-steroids-eczema/.

3. Attila Oláh et al., "Cannabidiol Exerts Sebostatic and Antiinflammatory Effects on Human Sebocytes," *The Journal of Clinical Investigation* 124, no. 9 (2014): 3713–3724.
4. Attila Oláh et al., "Differential Effectiveness of Selected Non-Psychotropic Phytocannabinoids on Human Sebocyte Functions Implicates Their Introduction in Dry/Seborrhoeic Skin and Acne Treatment," *Experimental Dermatology* 25, no. 9 (2016): 701–707.
5. Alif Ali and Naveed Akhtar, "The Safety and Efficacy of 3% Cannabis Seeds Extract Cream for Reduction of Human Cheek Skin Sebum and Erythema Content," *Pakistan Journal of Pharmaceutical Sciences* 28, no. 4 (2015): 1389–1395.
6. https://www.aad.org/media/news-releases/topical-cannabis.
7. John A. Karas et al., "The Antimicrobial Activity of Cannabinoids," *Antibiotics* 9, no. 7 (2020): 406.
8. Leon H. Kircik, "What's New in the Management of Acne Vulgaris," *Cutis* 104, no. 1 (2019): 48–52.
9. R. Dean Blevins and Michael P. Dumic, "The Effect of Δ-9-tetrahydrocannabinol on Herpes Simplex Virus Replication," *Journal of General Virology* 49, no. 2 (1980): 427–431; Maria M. Medveczky et al., "Delta-9-tetrahydrocannabinol (THC) Inhibits Lytic Replication of Gamma Oncogenic Herpesviruses in Vitro," *BMC Medicine* 2, no. 1 (2004): 1–9.
10. https://www.aafa.org/media/2209/Atopic-Dermatitis-in-America-Study-Overview.pdf.
11. Jon M. Hanifin and Michael L. Reed, Eczema Prevalence and Impact Working Group, "A Population-based Survey of Eczema Prevalence in the United States," *Dermatitis* 18, no. 2 (2007): 82–91.
12. Giovanni Appendino et al., "Antibacterial Cannabinoids from Cannabis Sativa: A Structure-Activity Study," *Journal of Natural Products* 71, no. 8 (2008): 1427–1430.
13. Balvindra Singh, Nazma Haque, and Neelam Singh, "Nosocomial Infections: Anti-MRSA Activity of Cannabis Sativa and THUJA Orientalis Active Components Obtained by TLC," *International Journal of Recent Scientific Research* 10, no. 4 (2019): 31933–31937.
14. Appendino et al., "Antibacterial Cannabinoids."
15. https://nationaleczema.org/can-marijuana-help/.
16. April W. Armstrong et al., "Real-world Utilization Patterns of Systemic Immunosuppressants among US Adult Patients with Atopic Dermatitis," *PLOS ONE* 14, no. 1 (2019): e0210517.
17. Armstrong et al., "Real-world Utilization."
18. Henry Granger Piffard, *A Treatise on the Materia Medica and Therapeutics of the Skin* (W. Wood, 1881), https://nationaleczema.org/can-marijuana-help/.

19. Jessica S. Mounessa et al., “The Role of Cannabinoids in Dermatology,” *Journal of the American Academy of Dermatology* 77, no. 1 (2017): 188–190.
20. https://www.skintherapyletter.com/dermatology/cannabinoids-potential/.
21. https://nationaleczema.org/eczema-emotional-wellness/.
22. https://nationaleczema.org/eczema-emotional-wellness/.
23. https://www.psoriasis.org/psoriatic-arthritis.
24. Nima Derakhshan and Mahboubeh Kazemi, “Cannabis for Refractory Psoriasis—High Hopes for a Novel Treatment and a Literature Review,” *Current Clinical Pharmacology* 11, no. 2 (2016): 146–147.
25. https://www.medicalnewstoday.com/articles/320086.php.
26. Jonathan D. Wilkinson and Elizabeth M. Williamson, “Cannabinoids Inhibit Human Keratinocyte Proliferation through a Non-CB1/CB2 Mechanism and Have a Potential Therapeutic Value in the Treatment of Psoriasis,” *Journal of Dermatological Science* 45, no. 2 (2007): 87–92.
27. Shan-Shan Li et al., “Cannabinoid CB2 Receptors Are Involved in the Regulation of Fibrogenesis during Skin Wound Repair in Mice,” *Molecular Medicine Reports* 13, no. 4 (2016): 3441–3450.
28. Adam J. Friedman, Kimia Momeni, and Mikhail Kogan, “Topical Cannabinoids for the Management of Psoriasis Vulgaris: Report of a Case and Review of the Literature,” *Journal of Drugs in Dermatology: JDD* 19, no. 8 (2020): 795.
29. https://www.alliedmarketresearch.com/cbd-skin-care-market.
30. Marcel O. Bonn-Miller et al., “Labeling Accuracy of Cannabidiol Extracts Sold Online,” *JAMA* 318, no. 17 (2017): 1708–1709.
31. Atif Ali, “Phenolics for Skin Photo-aging,” *Pakistan Journal of Pharmaceutical Sciences* 30, no. 4 (2017).
32. https://www.skincancer.org/skin-cancer-information/skin-cancer-facts/.
33. Jane L. Armstrong et al., “Exploiting Cannabinoid-induced Cytotoxic Autophagy to Drive Melanoma Cell Death,” *Journal of Investigative Dermatology* 135, no. 6 (2015): 1629–1637; Ava Bachari et al., “Roles of Cannabinoids in Melanoma: Evidence from In Vivo Studies,” *International Journal of Molecular Sciences* 21, no. 17 (2020): 6040.

CHAPTER 8: CANCER

1. Amber S. Kleckner et al., “Opportunities for Cannabis in Supportive Care in Cancer,” *Therapeutic Advances in Medical Oncology* 11 (2019): 1–29.
2. Steven A. Pergam et al., “Cannabis Use among Patients at a Comprehensive Cancer Center in a State with Legalized Medicinal and Recreational Use,” *Cancer* 123, no. 22 (2017): 4488–4497; Kevin Martell et al., “Rates of Cannabis Use in Patients with Cancer,” *Current Oncology* 25, no. 3 (2018): 219–225.
3. Donald Abrams, email to Mikhail Kogan, November 6, 2020.

4. https://www.cancer.gov/about-cancer/treatment/side-effects/nausea/nausea-hp-pdq.
5. Megan Brafford May and Ashley E. Glode, "Dronabinol for Chemotherapy-induced Nausea and Vomiting Unresponsive to Antiemetics," *Cancer Management and Research* 8 (2016): 49.
6. Karen M. Mustian et al., "Treatment of Nausea and Vomiting during Chemotherapy," *US Oncology & Hematology* 7, no. 2 (2011): 91.
7. https://www.cancer.gov/about-cancer/treatment/side-effects/nausea/nausea-pdq.
8. Yolanda Escobar et al., "Incidence of Chemotherapy-induced Nausea and Vomiting with Moderately Emetogenic Chemotherapy: ADVICE (Actual Data of Vomiting Incidence by Chemotherapy Evaluation) Study," *Supportive Care in Cancer* 23, no. 9 (2015): 2833–2840.
9. Escobar et al., "Incidence of Chemotherapy-induced Nausea and Vomiting."
10. Keith A. Sharkey and John W. Wiley, "The Role of the Endocannabinoid System in the Brain-Gut Axis," *Gastroenterology* 151, no. 2 (2016): 252–266.
11. National Academies of Sciences, Engineering, and Medicine, "The Health Effects of Cannabis and Cannabinoids: The Current State of Evidence and Recommendations for Research," (2017), 94, https://www.ncbi.nlm.nih.gov/books/NBK425767/.
12. Melissa E. Badowski, "A Review of Oral Cannabinoids and Medical Marijuana for the Treatment of Chemotherapy-induced Nausea and Vomiting: A Focus on Pharmacokinetic Variability and Pharmacodynamics," *Cancer Chemotherapy and Pharmacology* 80, no. 3 (2017): 441–449.
13. May, "Dronabinol for Chemotherapy"; Badowski, "A Review of Oral Cannabinoids"; Young D. Chang et al., "Edmonton Symptom Assessment Scale and Clinical Characteristics Associated with Cannabinoid Use in Oncology Supportive Care Outpatients," *Journal of the National Comprehensive Cancer Network* 17, no. 9 (2019): 1059–1064.
14. May, "Dronabinol for Chemotherapy."
15. Mikhail Kogan and Michelle Sexton, *Medical Cannabis: A New Old Tool for Palliative Care, The Journal of Alternative and Complementary Medicine* 26, no. 9 (2020): 778–780.
16. Chang, "Edmonton Symptom Assessment Scale."
17. Joan L. Kramer, "Medical Marijuana for Cancer," *CA: A Cancer Journal for Clinicians* 65, no. 2 (2015): 109–122.
18. May, "Dronabinol for Chemotherapy."
19. Janet Joy and Alison Mack, *Marijuana as Medicine?: The Science beyond the Controversy*, The National Academies of Sciences, Engineering, and Medicine (Washington, DC: National Academies Press, 2000), 100–101.
20. Kleckner, "Opportunities for Cannabis."
21. Robert L. Page et al., "Medical Marijuana, Recreational Cannabis, and Cardiovascular Health: A Scientific Statement from the American Heart As-

sociation," *Circulation* 142, no. 10 (2020): e131–e152. https://www.heart.org/en/news/2020/08/05/heart-risks-of-marijuana-use-need-more-research.

22. Pergam, "Cannabis Use among Patients."
23. D. I. Abrams, "Integrating Cannabis into Clinical Cancer Care," *Current Oncology* 23, Suppl 2 (2016): S8; Sonia A. Tucci, "Phytochemicals in the Control of Human Appetite and Body Weight," *Pharmaceuticals* 3, no. 3 (2010): 748–763.
24. Donald I. Abrams et al., "Cannabis in Painful HIV-associated Sensory Neuropathy: A Randomized Placebo-controlled Trial," *Neurology* 68, no. 7 (2007): 515–521; Kramer, "Medical Marijuana for Cancer."
25. T. D. Brisbois et al., "Delta-9-tetrahydrocannabinol May Palliate Altered Chemosensory Perception in Cancer Patients: Results of a Randomized, Double-Blind, Placebo-Controlled Pilot Trial," *Annals of Oncology* 22, no. 9 (2011): 2086–2093.
26. Jennifer Cohen, Claire E. Wakefield, and David G. Laing, "Smell and Taste Disorders Resulting from Cancer and Chemotherapy," *Current Pharmaceutical Design* 22, no. 15 (2016): 2253–2263.
27. Mikhail Kogan, ed., *Integrative Geriatric Medicine* (New York: Oxford University Press, 2017).
28. Andrea M. Tomko et al., "Anti-Cancer Potential of Cannabinoids, Terpenes, and Flavonoids Present in Cannabis," *Cancers* 12, no. 7 (2020): 1985.
29. Olga Kovalchuk and Igor Kovalchuk, "Cannabinoids as Anticancer Therapeutic Agents," *Cell Cycle* 19, no. 9 (2020): 961–989.
30. American Cancer Society. "Special Section: Cancer-Related Pain," *Cancer Facts & Figures 2007.* Atlanta: American Cancer Society; 2007. https://www.cancer.org/content/dam/cancer-org/research/cancer-facts-and-statistics/annual-cancer-facts-and-figures/2007/special-section-cancer-facts-and-figures-2007.pdf.
31. Marieke H. J. van den Beuken-van Everdingen et al., "Update on Prevalence of Pain in Patients with Cancer: Systematic Review and Meta-Analysis," *Journal of Pain and Symptom Management* 51, no. 6 (2016): 1070–1090.
32. https://www.nccn.org/patients/resources/life_with_cancer/managing_symptoms/neuropathy.aspx.
33. Janice N. Cormier et al., "Lymphedema beyond Breast Cancer: A Systematic Review and Meta-Analysis of Cancer-Related Secondary Lymphedema," *Cancer* 116, no. 22 (2010): 5138–5149.
34. Matthew R. D. Brown, Juan D. Ramirez, and Paul Farquhar-Smith, "Pain in Cancer Survivors," *British Journal of Pain* 8, no. 4 (2014): 139–153.
35. Yuval Zolotov, Lia Eshet, and Ofir Morag, "Preliminary Assessment of Medical Cannabis Consumption by Cancer Survivors," *Complementary Therapies in Medicine* 56 (2021): 102592.
36. https://www.ascopost.com/issues/september-15-2013/undertreatment-of-cancer-pain-remains-a-persistent-problem-in-oncology/.
37. https://www.cancer.org/treatment/treatments-and-side-effects/physical-side-effects/pain/opioid-pain-medicines-for-cancer-pain.html.

38. Paula Parás-Bravo et al., "Association among Presence of Cancer Pain, Inadequate Pain Control, and Psychotropic Drug Use," *PLOS ONE* 12, no. 6 (2017): e0178742; https://www.ascopost.com/issues/september-15-2013/undertreatment-of-cancer-pain-remains-a-persistent-problem-in-oncology/.
39. https://www.cancer.gov/about-cancer/treatment/cam/hp/cannabis-pdq.
40. Alexia Blake et al., "A Selective Review of Medical Cannabis in Cancer Pain Management," *Annals of Palliative Medicine* 6, Suppl 2 (2017): s215–s222; Amber S. Kleckner et al., "Opportunities for Cannabis in Supportive Care in Cancer," *Therapeutic Advances in Medical Oncology* 11 (2019): 1758835919866362.
41. Jeremy R. Johnson et al., "Multicenter, Double-Blind, Randomized, Placebo-Controlled, Parallel-Group Study of the Efficacy, Safety, and Tolerability of THC:CBD Extract and THC Extract in Patients with Intractable Cancer-Related Pain," *Journal of Pain and Symptom Management* 39, no. 2 (2010): 167–179.
42. https://www.ancient-origins.net/news-history-archaeology/did-ancient-siberian-princess-use-cannabis-cope-breast-cancer-002207.
43. Barth Wilsey et al., "Low-Dose Vaporized Cannabis Significantly Improves Neuropathic Pain," *The Journal of Pain* 14, no. 2 (2013): 136–148; Abrams, "Cannabis in Painful HIV."
44. Abrams, "Integrating Cannabis."
45. Ian Pawasarat et al., "The Efficacy of Medical Marijuana in the Treatment of Cancer-Related Pain," *Journal of Palliative Medicine* 23, no. 6 (2020): 809–816.
46. Sharad Goyal Sindhu Kubendran, Mikhail Kogan, and Yuan J. Rao, "High Expectations: The Landscape of Clinical Trials of Medical Marijuana in Oncology," *Complementary Therapies in Medicine* 49 (2020): 102336.
47. Kleckner, "Opportunities for Cannabis."
48. Abrams, "Integrating Cannabis."
49. Lihi Bar-Lev Schleider et al., "Prospective Analysis of Safety and Efficacy of Medical Cannabis in Large Unselected Population of Patients with Cancer," *European Journal of Internal Medicine* 49 (2018): 37–43; Erin A. Blake et al., "Non-Prescription Cannabis Use for Symptom Management Amongst Women with Gynecologic Malignancies," *Gynecologic Oncology Reports* 30 (2019): 100497; Deanna Teoh et al., "Care after Chemotherapy: Peripheral Neuropathy, Cannabis for Symptom Control, and Mindfulness," *American Society of Clinical Oncology Educational Book* 38 (2018): 469–479.
50. Zolotov, "Preliminary Assessment."
51. Marcus A. Bachhuber et al., "Medical Cannabis Laws and Opioid Analgesic Overdose Mortality in the United States, 1999–2010," *JAMA Internal Medicine* 174, no. 10 (2014): 1668–1673.
52. Mikhail Kogan, ed., *Integrative Geriatric Medicine* (New York: Oxford University Press, 2017).

53. S. K. Aggarwal, "Use of Cannabinoids in Cancer Care: Palliative Care," *Current Oncology* 23, Suppl 2 (2016): 3.
54. Goyal et al., "High Expectations."
55. Pawel Śledziński et al., "The Current State and Future Perspectives of Cannabinoids in Cancer Biology," *Cancer Medicine* 7, no. 3 (2018): 765–775.
56. Abrams, "Integrating Cannabis," 511.
57. Ava Bachari et al., "Roles of Cannabinoids in Melanoma: Evidence from In Vivo Studies," *International Journal of Molecular Sciences* 21, no. 17 (2020): 6040.
58. Bachari et al., "Roles of Cannabinoids in Melanoma," 3.
59. Donald I. Abrams and Manuel Guzmán, "Can Cannabis Cure Cancer?," *JAMA Oncology* 6, no. 3 (2020): 323–324.
60. Abrams and Guzmán, "Can Cannabis Cure Cancer?"
61. B. Polushaj and M. Kogan, "Do You Know Where Your Patient's Cannabis Comes From? Dramatic Response to Integrative Treatment in Patient with Stage IV Colon Cancer," poster, 2018 International Congress on Integrative Medicine & Health and Academic Consortium for Integrative Health and Medicine Annual Meeting, May 8–11, 2018, Baltimore, MD.
62. Abrams and Guzmán, "Can Cannabis Cure Cancer?"; Śledziński, "The Current State."
63. Tomko, "Anti-Cancer Potential."
64. Brigitta Kis et al., "Cannabidiol—From Plant to Human Body: A Promising Bioactive Molecule with Multi-Target Effects in Cancer," *International Journal of Molecular Sciences* 20, no. 23 (2019): 5905.

CHAPTER 9: CHRONIC NEUROLOGICAL CONDITIONS

1. Daniel M. Hartung, "Economics and Cost-Effectiveness of Multiple Sclerosis Therapies in the USA," *Neurotherapeutics* 14, no. 4 (2017): 1018–1026.
2. https://www.cando-ms.org/online-resources/can-do-library/cannabis-for-multiple-sclerosis-symptoms.
3. John H. Kindred et al., "Cannabis Use in People with Parkinson's Disease and Multiple Sclerosis: A Web-Based Investigation," *Complementary Therapies in Medicine* 33 (2017): 99–104.
4. Kindred et al., "Cannabis Use in People."
5. K. P. Hill, "Medical Marijuana for Treatment of Chronic Pain and Other Medical and Psychiatric Problems: A Clinical Review," *JAMA* 313, no. 24 (2015): 2474.
6. M. A. Mecha et al., "Cannabidiol and Multiple Sclerosis," in *Handbook of Cannabis and Related Pathologies* (Cambridge, MA: Academic Press, 2017), 893–904; Thorsten Rudroff and Jacob Sosnoff, "Cannabidiol to Improve Mobility in People with Multiple Sclerosis," *Frontiers in Neurology* 9 (2018): 183.

7. Laura Weinkle et al., "Exploring Cannabis Use by Patients with Multiple Sclerosis in a State Where Cannabis Is Legal," *Multiple Sclerosis and Related Disorders* 27 (2019): 383–390.
8. Nancy Maurya and Bharath Kumar Velmurugan, "Therapeutic Applications of Cannabinoids," *Chemico-Biological Interactions* 293 (2018): 77–88.
9. Kindred, "Cannabis Use in People."
10. J. B. Guarnaccia et al., "Patterns of Medical Cannabis Use among Patients Diagnosed with Multiple Sclerosis," *Multiple Sclerosis and Related Disorders* (2021): 102830.
11. https://www.michaeljfox.org/causes.
12. https://medlineplus.gov/genetics/condition/parkinson-disease/.
13. https://www.parkinson.org/understanding-parkinsons/causes/genetics.
14. Rikinkumar S. Patel et al., "Pros and Cons of Marijuana in Treatment of Parkinson's Disease," *Cureus* 11, no. 6 (2019): e4813.
15. https://www.sciencedaily.com/releases/2020/05/200501150558.htm.
16. S. L. Wu et al., "Nonmotor Symptoms of Parkinson's Disease," *Parkinson's Disease* (2017): 4382518.
17. Antoniya Todorova, Peter Jenner, and K. Ray Chaudhuri, "Non-Motor Parkinson's: Integral to Motor Parkinson's, Yet Often Neglected," *Practical Neurology* 14, no. 5 (2014): 310–322.
18. https://www.parkinson.org/Understanding-Parkinsons/Treatment/Medical-Marijuana.
19. Christopher G. Goetz, "The History of Parkinson's Disease: Early Clinical Descriptions and Neurological Therapies," *Cold Spring Harbor Perspectives in Medicine* 1, no. 1 (2011): a008862.
20. W. R. Gowers, *A Manual of Diseases of the Nervous System*, Vol. 1 (P. Blakiston's Sons & Company, 1896). https://www.projectcbd.org/medicine/cbd-and-parkinsons-disease.
21. Mariana Babayeva et al., "Marijuana Compounds: A Nonconventional Approach to Parkinson's Disease Therapy," *Parkinson's Disease* 2016 (2016); Mario Stampanoni Bassi et al., "Cannabinoids in Parkinson's Disease," *Cannabis and Cannabinoid Research* 2, no. 1 (2017): 21–29; Kateřina Venderová et al., "Survey on Cannabis Use in Parkinson's Disease: Subjective Improvement of Motor Symptoms," *Movement Disorders* 19, no. 9 (2004): 1102–1106.
22. Taylor Andrew Finseth et al., "Self-Reported Efficacy of Cannabis and Other Complementary Medicine Modalities by Parkinson's Disease Patients in Colorado," *Evidence-Based Complementary and Alternative Medicine* 2015 (2015); Yacov Balash et al., "Medical Cannabis in Parkinson Disease: Real-Life Patients' Experience," *Clinical Neuropharmacology* 40, no. 6 (2017): 268–272; A. A. Shohet et al., "Effect of Medical Cannabis on Thermal Quantitative Measurements of Pain in Patients with Parkinson's Disease," *European Journal of Pain* 21, no. 3 (2017): 486–493.

23. Kindred, "Cannabis Use in People."
24. https://www.alz.org/media/documents/alzheimers-facts-and-figures-2019-r.pdf.
25. Uma Suryadevara et al., "Pros and Cons of Medical Cannabis Use by People with Chronic Brain Disorders," *Current Neuropharmacology* 15, no. 6 (2017): 800–814.
26. Nathan Herrmann et al., "Randomized Placebo-Controlled Trial of Nabilone for Agitation in Alzheimer's Disease," *The American Journal of Geriatric Psychiatry* 27, no. 11 (2019): 1161–1173.
27. Konstantina G. Yiannopoulou et al., "Reasons for Failed Trials of Disease-Modifying Treatments for Alzheimer Disease and Their Contribution in Recent Research," *Biomedicines* 7, no. 4 (2019): 97.
28. https://www.aarp.org/content/dam/aarp/ppi/2018/08/reducing-potential-overuse-of-dementia-drugs-could-lead-to-considerable-savings.pdf.
29. https://www.aarp.org/content/dam/aarp/ppi/2018/04/off-label-antipsychotic-use-in-older-adults-with-dementia.pdf.
30. https://www.aarp.org/content/dam/aarp/ppi/2018/04/off-label-antipsychotic-use-in-older-adults-with-dementia.pdf.
31. Yiannopoulou, "Reasons for Failed Trials."
32. Ethan B. Russo, "Cannabis Therapeutics and the Future of Neurology," *Frontiers in Integrative Neuroscience* 12 (2018): 51.
33. Suryadevara, "Pros and Cons."
34. https://www.salk.edu/news-release/cannabinoids-remove-plaque-forming-alzheimers-proteins-from-brain-cells/
35. Suryadevara, "Pros and Cons."
36. Suryadevara, "Pros and Cons."
37. Herrmann, "Randomized Placebo-Controlled Trial."
38. www.goodrx.com.
39. Russo, "Cannabis Therapeutics."
40. Assaf Shelef et al., "Safety and Efficacy of Medical Cannabis Oil for Behavioral and Psychological Symptoms of Dementia: An Open-Label, Add-On, Pilot Study," *Journal of Alzheimer's Disease* 51, no. 1 (2016): 15–19.
41. Barbara Broers et al., "Prescription of a THC/CBD-Based Medication to Patients with Dementia: A Pilot Study in Geneva," *Medical Cannabis and Cannabinoids* 2, no. 1 (2019): 56–59.
42. Russo, "Cannabis Therapeutics."
43. Kwakye Peprah and Suzanne McCormack, "Medical Cannabis for the Treatment of Dementia: A Review of Clinical Effectiveness and Guidelines," Canadian Agency for Drugs and Technologies in Health, Ottawa (2019), 12.
44. Mikhail Kogan and Michelle Sexton, "Medical Cannabis: A New Old Tool for Palliative Care," *The Journal of Alternative and Complementary Medicine* 26, no. 9 (2020): 778–780.

45. D. E. Bredesen et al., "Reversal of Cognitive Decline: 100 Patients," *The Journal of Alzheimer's Disease & Parkinsonism* 8, no. 450 (2018). https://www.researchgate.net/publication/329063941_Reversal_of_Cognitive_Decline_100_Patients.
46. Madeline M. Foley et al., "One Man's Swordfish Story: The Link between Alzheimer's Disease and Mercury Exposure," *Complementary Therapies in Medicine* 52 (2020): 102499.
47. Kogan and Sexton, "Medical Cannabis."

CHAPTER 10: DEALING WITH DOCTORS AND DISPENSARIES

1. Kevin F. Boehnke et al., "Qualifying Conditions of Medical Cannabis License Holders in the United States," *Health Affairs* 38, no. 2 (2019): 295–302.
2. https://www.marijuanadoctors.com/medical-marijuana/il/qualification/.
3. https://www.medpagetoday.com/infectiousdisease/covid19/86254?vpass=1.
4. Elin C. Kondrad et al., "Lack of Communication about Medical Marijuana Use between Doctors and Their Patients," *The Journal of the American Board of Family Medicine* 31, no. 5 (2018): 805–808.
5. Lindsey M. Philpot, Jon O. Ebbert, and Ryan T. Hurt, "A Survey of the Attitudes, Beliefs and Knowledge about Medical Cannabis among Primary Care Providers," *BMC Family Practice* 20, no. 1 (2019): 1–7; Rita Rubin, "Medical Marijuana Is Legal in Most States, but Physicians Have Little Evidence to Guide Them," *JAMA* 317, no. 16 (2017): 1611–1613.
6. Kevin M. Takakuwa et al., "Education, Knowledge, and Practice Characteristics of Cannabis Physicians: A Survey of the Society of Cannabis Clinicians," *Cannabis and Cannabinoid Research* 6, no. 1, (2021): 58–65.
7. https://www.safeaccessnow.org/travel.
8. https://wayofleaf.com/blog/can-you-cross-state-lines-with-marijuana.
9. https://www.safeaccessnow.org/travel.
10. https://travel.gc.ca/travelling/cannabis-and-international-travel.
11. https://www.roadaffair.com/traveling-with-cannabis.
12. https://www.newsamericasnow.com/how-do-dispensaries-get-weed-to-sell/.
13. https://www.safeaccessnow.org/iqa_victory.
14. https://www.leafly.com/news/cannabis-101/how-to-read-cannabis-product-label.
15. Cesar Leos-Toro et al., "Cannabis Labeling and Consumer Understanding of THC Levels and Serving Sizes," *Drug and Alcohol Dependence* 208 (2020): 107843.
16. https://dfcr.org/.
17. D. L. Nathan, "Setting the Standard for Cannabis Labeling: Introducing the Universal Cannabis Product Symbol and the Universal Cannabis

Information Label," *Cannabis Science and Technology* 3, no. 6 (2020): 44–52. https://dfcr.org/setting-the-standard-for-cannabis-labeling/.
18. Nathan, "Setting the Standard for Cannabis Labeling," 44.
19. https://www.safeaccessnow.org/asa_medical_marijuana_policy_position.
20. https://www.prnewswire.com/news-releases/americans-for-safe-access-unveils-2019-report-cards-for-medical-cannabis-programs-across-the-us-300897607.html.
21. https://www.practicalpainmanagement.com/patient/treatments/marijuana-cannabis/two-surveys-show-what-consumers-know-about-cannabis.
22. https://www.verywellhealth.com/why-health-insurance-wont-pay-for-medical-marijuana-1738421?print.
23. https://www.verywellhealth.com/why-health-insurance-wont-pay-for-medical-marijuana-1738421?print.
24. https://docmj.com/2019/12/09/whats-the-difference-between-marinol-medical-marijuana/.
25. https://wayofleaf.com/blog/buy-high-quality-weed-discount-price; https://www.leafly.com/brands/your-weed-coupons.
26. Nancy A. Haug et al., "Training and Practices of Cannabis Dispensary Staff," *Cannabis and Cannabinoid Research* 1, no. 1 (2016): 244–251.
27. Roberto Linares et al., "Personnel Training and Patient Education in Medical Marijuana Dispensaries in Oregon," *Journal of the American Pharmacists Association* 56, no. 3 (2016): 270–273.
28. Rubin, "Medical Marijuana Is Legal in Most States," 1612.
29. Leslie Mendoza Temple, Sara L. Lampert, and Bernard Ewigman, "Barriers to Achieving Optimal Success with Medical Cannabis: Opportunities for Quality Improvement," *The Journal of Alternative and Complementary Medicine* 25, no. 1 (2019): 6.
30. https://mmcc.maryland.gov/Pages/Clinical-Directors.aspx.
31. Linares, "Personnel Training and Patient Education."
32. Temple, "Barriers to Achieving Optimal Success."
33. Takakuwa, "Education, Knowledge, and Practice."
34. https://www.journals.elsevier.com/complementary-therapies-in-medicine/call-for-papers/call-for-papers-medical-cannabis-in-professional-education.
35. Temple, "Barriers to Achieving Optimal Success."
36. Rubin, "Medical Marijuana Is Legal in Most States."

Index